ALZHEIMER'S –
LIFE IN REVERSE

By
Dr. Philip C Minter, A M

ISBN 10: 1503015580
LCCN: 2014919353

CreateSpace Independent Publishing Platform
North Charleston, South Carolina

ISBN 13:978-1503015586

FOREWORD

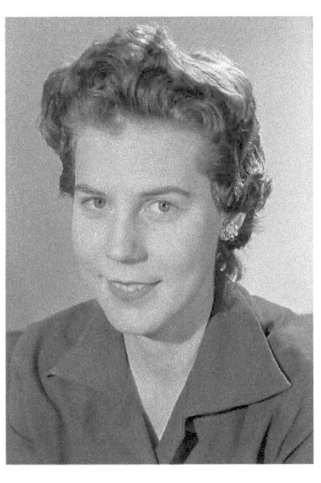

Was it love at first sight when Philip Minter met Mary Schettler?

Most likely - after all, they were married after a four-month courtship! It was a whirlwind romance - that lasted more than 40 years.

The title of this book - **Alzheimer's, Life in Reverse** - may not sound like a love story, but as any Alzheimer's family will tell you, the disease tests your love like nothing else.

At first Philip and Mary had a life to be admired, perhaps even envied. They were an international couple, successful entrepreneurs with a fulfilling family life. It was a life many who knew them may have even secretly wanted to duplicate. They travelled extensively on three continents, one daughter born in Australia, another born in Colorado. They finally settled in Philadelphia and spent most of their married life in the United States.

Life was non-stop, full steam ahead, until one day the family began to notice that Mary was not performing to her usual high standards. She was forgetting details at work and home, not following through with projects, so much so that she had to stop working in the family business. One evening at a social gathering a doctor whispered to Philip - Alzheimer's.

What's that?

Philip and his daughters learned they were dealing with Early Onset Alzheimer's - a rare and aggressive form of the disease that usually strikes people in their forties and fifties. Mary was only 54!

They also quickly realized they were watching "Life in Reverse". A child is on a learning curve, going from requiring 100% care and attention to 100% independence. But with Alzheimer's, the adult regresses, losing abilities until they reach a stage of needing 100% care and attention, 100% supervision around the clock, and losing all independence. They must rely on a loving caregiver to see to their every need.

This is a very personal, no-holds-barred story, of how a normal life, perhaps upper middle class, of careers, church, daughters graduating from college, social activities, travel, gets turned upside down by this insidious disease.

It is a detailed, and frankly sometimes disturbing account of their experience with the disease, the testing Mary went through, the clinical trials they participated in, the difficult decision to move to a nursing home and the challenges and agonies that followed.

Nothing in life prepares you for Alzheimer's; there is no immunity, no prevention, and no cure.

Nothing can prepare the patient or caregiver for what the disease brings as it progresses.

As of this publication, it is estimated that there are more than 5 million Americans living with Alzheimer's and more than 15 million caregivers, mainly close family members, attending to them around the clock.

Caregivers can help one another by sharing their stories; Dr. Philip Minter has done just that.

James A. Cassidy

Cassidy was a caregiver to his wife, also named Mary, also a victim of Early Onset Alzheimer's Disease; He served as the General Manager of The Monitor newspaper for the Diocese of Trenton in NJ, and served on the Board of Directors for the Catholic Advertising Network. Cassidy also served as editor for this book.

"…Dr. Minter clearly loved his wife and has written about their experience with Alzheimer's disease as a way of honoring her spirit. His accounts of their life are touching and tender. When she is in a nursing home, he depicts accurately the complexities of negotiating with the patient (bathing, eating), with the staff (management of illness, falls), and other residents (men pushing his wife and how this is handled). It reads like a journal and remains a factual account of Mary's existence, pre and post illness.

This is a heartfelt attempt to share a family's experience with a devastating disease. It takes courage to write a book such as this and I applaud Dr. Minter's efforts. There is a lot of material here worth exploring, and is an important and worthwhile endeavor that I know families affected by AD will value…"

Felicia Greenfield,
Associate Director for Clinical and Research Operations
Penn Memory Center

ALZHEIMER'S – LIFE IN REVERSE
CONTENTS

LIFE IN WISCONSIN…

CHAPTER 1

WHO WAS MARY MINTER?

On December 30, 1933, Mary Bashford Schettler was born in Madison, Wisconsin, the second child of Franklin and Violet Schettler of Beaver Dam, Wisconsin.

She was a bright, well loved woman who came to maturity in the immediate post-war years, when many say American culture reached its zenith. She was overtaken by senile dementia at a relatively young age. She was also my wife.

By learning who Mary was and the influence of her early years, you may come to understand the tragedy of her final years. Her high level of intelligence and broad life-time experience may have contributed to the very slow decline she experienced from the time she was first diagnosed as suffering from Alzheimer's disease.

Mary was truly a member of the American middle class. She was a college graduate with a mid-western accent who had traveled to a limited extent in her early years and worldwide as an adult. She was a member of a close-knit, but not extensive family who had grown up with a small core of friends in a small mid-western town.

Her parents were both first generation Americans, born in the last decade of the nineteenth century. Her mother, Violet, whose parents had arrived in Wisconsin from London, attended a junior college and was a primary school teacher prior to her marriage. It was somewhat unusual for English families to settle in Wisconsin where the population tended to be of German, Swiss, Norwegian or Polish ancestry. Perhaps that was why Violet and her sister Ruth came to be ardent Anglophiles, even though one married a German and the other a Swiss. Mary's father graduated from high school and joined the U.S. Army during World War I. He became a sergeant, but was not sent overseas.

Mary's grandparents on her father's side were from Berlin, Germany. After arriving in Wisconsin, her grandfather had built a business that made wagon wheels. Naturally, that business fell into decline with the advent of automobiles and trucks. Following World War I, her father joined the Malleable Iron Range Company in Beaver Dam and became their credit manager. The Malleable Iron Range Company built Monarch Stoves, a premium line of, at first wood and coal, then later gas and electric stoves. Competition from multinational companies led to closure of that company in the 1980s.

Mary's parents were Republican and Episcopalian. It was said that Mary grew up thinking Franklin Roosevelt's first name was "God Damn". Both parents belonged to Masonic organizations. Franklin was a Shriner and Violet belonged to the Eastern Star. At an appropriate age, Mary joined "Job's Daughters" which is the Masonic organization for girls. She rose to the position of "honor queen" for the Beaver Dam Chapter. After college, she moved up to Eastern Star.

Mary had one sibling, a brother Bill. Being five years older than Mary, Bill had his own circle of friends, but remained close to Mary until he moved away to college and then joined the U.S. Navy.

Mary's parents had a hard attitude to sickness. It was clear in the Schettler family that sickness was considered an indication of weakness and a mental sickness especially was a moral weakness. The fact that Roosevelt had polio only strengthened their opinion of his unsuitability as President. A person who was sick and looking for sympathy was crudely called a "panty waster". Mary was almost never given any drugs or medications, except an occasional aspirin. The only childhood disease she contracted seemed to have been measles. The family attitude was hard, but did not seem to adversely affect Mary. It was prophetic that the family should have had this intolerant attitude to sickness and then the mother, father and daughter all developed what is arguably the most terrible form of mental degeneration.

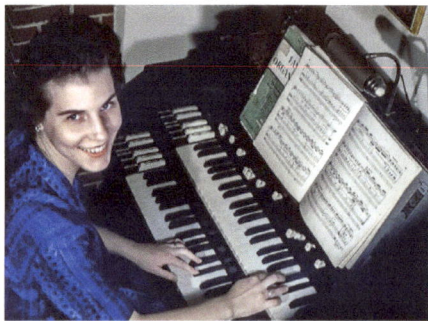

While her parents were not wealthy they managed their money well and made a good living. Prior to marriage, Mary's mother had taught school. After marriage, she devoted her time to her home and a few charities including the women's club. In the

1930s and 40s, wives of business executives did not work away from the home. Very soon after marrying, the Schettlers built a modest English Tudor style home on a corner lot about a half mile from the business section of town. Over the years, the home was beautifully decorated with a number of high quality Oriental rugs and comfortable furniture. A small Steinway piano was bought for Bill, and a church sized Hammond Organ was given to Mary. She learned to play both instruments. She was sufficiently skilled as an organist to occasionally play for her church.

Beaver Dam was a town of about 30,000 in the 1940s. The population remained somewhat the same in the 21st century. It was typical of hundreds of mid-western towns. There was a central business area, shops, and professional offices. As one moved out from the downtown center there were homes on fairly small lots. Further out there were several factories, a small railroad station and a bus depot. And, above all, there was a range of churches, although there was no synagogue, and the few Jewish families who did live in the town had to go to Milwaukee or Madison on holy days.

Many farms were located within a mile or so of the town center, while others were further away. Farm families used the town as their trading center while the upper middle class families of the town treated Madison and Chicago as their cultural centers. Most families in Beaver Dam subscribed to the Madison paper and the Chicago Tribune. The cultural organization of Middle America of the 1950s was different from the modern suburbia of present day America. Within the city limits of Beaver Dam, homes were on one quarter to half acre lots on tree lined streets with neat sidewalks. Mail was delivered twice per day directly into a slot in the front door. It was not until one entered the rural area outside the city limit, that one saw the now all common road-side mail box. At that time there was no such thing as a housing development on the outskirts of the town center of these mid-western towns.

Like many children at the time Mary could walk to school. She once mentioned that her IQ had been tested at 140 which is obviously a high average. Because she was bright, she scored good grades, although she did not have to work particularly hard. She participated in the cultural activities of Beaver Dam, such as art, music, and of course, Job's Daughters.

In addition to living well, her family kept up an image in Beaver Dam. By middle school years, it was decided that they would send Mary to Hillcrest, a small private girls school. Hillcrest was owned and managed by two elderly single women. According to Mary, the girls wore uniforms which were modified sailor suits. Some good friends she made at Hillcrest stayed in touch with her for the next 20 years.

In the summer of 1938, Mary's mother and her brother Bill went to England where Mrs. Schettler had cousins. Over the summer that her mother was away she spent much of the time with her aunt and uncle. In fact she usually spent much of every summer with her Aunt Ruth and Uncle Matt. Ruth was her mother's sister and had married a man of Swiss ancestry. They had no children so they lavished their love on Mary. Summer vacations were usually spent driving to Canada. Some years they went up through Duluth, along the north shores of Lake Superior to Port Arthur in Ontario. Then other years they drove over the upper peninsula of Michigan into Ontario then on to Montreal and Quebec. These were great vacations and Mary enjoyed them immensely. In fact she spoke of them up until she was no longer able to speak coherently.

Mary was eight when World War II started. The war was a primary developmental factor for all who grew up in the 1940s. While it is true that American children were not directly impacted by the war as were children in Great Britain or Europe, they were never-the-less affected by rationing and a general change in the social structure. There were not the gruesome scenes on TV as there were with the war in Vietnam - in fact there was no TV until after the war. There were however many things that impacted children such as the fact that there were few young men around and many families were in bereavement from the loss of sons or brothers. Mary's dad, who had served in World War I, became involved at his factory in the production of various items such as Jerry cans for the war effort.

Mary often talked about the Victory Garden that her father and uncle planted during those years and of course driving was restricted by gas rationing.

In addition to the Hillcrest School there is another private school in Beaver Dam, Wayland Academy, which was founded in 1840. It is a co-educational boarding school which, in the years when Mary attended, served largely as a school for wealthy children from Chicago. Mary's brother Bill had also attended Wayland. While it was primarily a boarding school both Mary and Bill attended as day students since they lived close by and were able to walk there. This school provided her with an excellent high school education and she maintained contact with her teachers even after she was married.

Mary graduated from Wayland in 1952 and was ready to go on to university. In the years following graduation, the president of Mary's class at Wayland continued to organize major reunions. The announcement for the 45th reunion arrived in November 1996, but we were unable to attend because Mary was then in a nursing home.

In the fall of 1952 Mary left home for the University of Wisconsin in Madison. Up to that time Mary had lived a sheltered and very up-scale existence but she elected not to enter a sorority. This was in line with her general attitude concerning elitist clubs or women's organizations. She would have nothing to do with organizations such as Eastern Star (after an initial bad experience), the Junior League, Daughters of the American Revolution, or P.E.O. (a secret organization of women). She considered that such groups were organized so that their members could feel elite and could criticize others outside their particular group. However, she did take an active role in a number of organizations which may be considered as being more egalitarian, including the American Women's Club in Australia, the American Association of University Women, and the Episcopal Church Women.

Mary entered Langdon Hall, a private dormitory where she met a number of girls who remained her friends in later life. Mary was certainly fond of men but often remarked how she would have hated to be in a coeducational dormitory. Such co-ed dormitories did not become popular until the 1960s. She said it would have been most restrictive to have men walking about when the women were going to the bathrooms and in casual clothes.

On entering the university she decided she wanted to become an interior decorator. The program for interior decorating at the University of Wisconsin was part of the Home Economics program called "Related Arts". The University campus is one of the major features of Madison which is also the state capital of Wisconsin. In the 1950s the enrollment was around 30,000. With students and faculty, the university contributed about half of the population of the city. At that time it was said that the university was one of the largest single items in the state budget.

The University of Wisconsin was absolutely a world class institution with a number of Nobel Laureates on the faculty. In biochemistry it was recognized as the world leader and other departments rated among the highest in the United States. I mention this academic excellence to which Mary was exposed because, while lower levels of education are thought to be a risk factor for developing Alzheimer's disease, it does not mean that people with higher levels of education will not develop the disease. Aside from Mary, I have known others suffering from Alzheimer's disease who attended major universities such as Harvard, Smith, Columbia, for example.

Madison, while at least 200 miles from a major city, never-the-less boasted excellent cultural opportunities. The theater at the Memorial Union attracted performers from all over the world. The city has warm humid summers and extremely cold winters. There may not be as much snow as in New England but it is certainly cold. On one morning in Mary's home town of Beaver Dam a temperature of 35 degrees below zero was recorded. That is 67 degrees below freezing. In the 1950s skiing was not a popular sport in Wisconsin and Mary never became a skier. Skiing may have became popular later, but the landscape is fairly flat and not particularly conducive to good down-hill skiing.

Mary seemed to have passed by most sporting activities which might have been available in other parts of the country but she did join the outdoors activity group called "Hoofers" and she became captain of the Archery team. Academically, Mary received a sound broad education with English, science classes, and a foreign language; Mary elected to take Italian. She was adequate but not brilliant and graduated Bachelor of Science in 1955.

CHAPTER 2

"AND SHE HAS A TURQUOISE THUNDERBIRD!"

These were the words with which I was first introduced to Mary Schettler.

After receiving a Master of Science Degree from the University of Wyoming, I decided to continue my studies towards a Ph.D. degree in Communications and I was accepted at the University of Wisconsin in Madison, in September 1958.

On several Sundays I attended the service at the Episcopal Student Center on the campus, and on one occasion, the chaplain asked me to give a talk on Australia on the second Sunday evening in October.

On those occasions students met in the library of the Student Center and then attended an Evensong Service. That was followed by a light supper and then some entertainment, such as a talk like mine, or games.

On my arrival, the chaplain, Rev. Gerald White, met me and said, "I would like you to meet one of our former students, Mary Schettler, who is visiting us this evening" He then leaned close and whispered, "and she has a turquoise Thunderbird!" I met Mary and we talked briefly. I admit to an immediate interest in her. She had a striking face, an interesting firm figure, 5 feet 6 inches and about 140 pounds. She seemed disinterested in my having recently arrived from Wyoming and she informed me that she was a decorator at a major Madison furniture store but was about to take a job at a leading department store in San Francisco. I remember wishing that she would stay around so I could get to know her better. We then walked into the chapel and sat together during the short service. Following graduation Mary had secured a position with Frautshi's Inc., the leading furniture store in Madison. She was employed as the store's first decorator and

9

worked on a small salary plus commission. Mary loved selecting the appropriate furniture and accessories for her clients but after she presented the plans she would sit back and let the customer decide whether to buy. Thus she was not a forceful salesperson and consequently seldom made much in commission. In fact she much preferred to work on commercial projects such as decorating the Madison Club and at another time taking the contract to decorate the Wisconsin Governor's Mansion. With industrial assignments she was able to design within the limits of the contracted budget and did not need to persuade someone that her ideas would look great, which they always did. Mary had a mild disposition with very nice tastes. She hated to have to press her opinion on others and this meant that most organizations found her non-threatening. This disposition led to her election to management roles in a number of organizations.

After getting the position in Madison, Mary rented a nice one bedroom apartment about 3 blocks from the Wisconsin Capital building and just a short walk to the furniture store. In this way she was able to sleep in until 9 a.m. and then reach the store by opening time at 9.30. Her next purchase was a car. Being a sophisticated lady, she decided on a Ford Thunderbird - the original 1955 model - in her favorite color – turquoise. The car certainly suited her personality.

During this time her mother persuaded Mary to join Eastern Star, the Masonic Women's Organization. Organizations such as this did not suit Mary's personality. While not a constant church-goer she did maintain a fairly close contact with the Episcopal Church. On the weekends when she returned home to Beaver Dam the family always attended the local church together. In Madison she occasionally attended the Episcopal Student Center, St. Francis House, where we first met.

After the service Mary sat with me during supper and she stayed after the talk to look at spears and boomerangs which I had out in my car. During the next week I thought about Mary a great deal and decided to go to the morning church service at St. Francis House the following week. Sure enough Mary was there also and we drifted together for coffee after the service. I took this opportunity to ask Mary if she would care to join me for lunch. She agreed. We went to the cafeteria at the University Union. There a funny thing happened. We filled our trays and as we went through the register, I was going to pay for both lunches. Mary said "Oh no, I will pay for mine you will have plenty of more opportunities to pay". Realizing what she had said, Mary went red and apologized. That afternoon I fixed a small problem with the Thunderbird; then we removed the top and went driving with the car as an open convertible - and it was late October in Wisconsin! The temperature was about freezing point.

Two weeks later, Mary asked me to visit her home for the Sunday. Unfortunately Mary was rather naive and had told her aunt Ruth that she had met the man she was going to marry, not expecting that her aunt would immediately phone her sister. Consequently I received a rather cool reception on my first visit to the Schettler home.

The next week end Mary suggested that we go to Chicago so she could show me the sights. We drove in the Thunderbird. This was quite an adventure. I had owned a rather sluggish pick-up truck in Australia and now had a 1953 Buick with Dynaflow transmission. With the Thunderbird I was able to spin the wheels by pushing the accelerator down while we were already doing 60 miles per hour. In Chicago we stayed at the Palmer House.

You may be surprised at how puritanical the American culture was in 1958. After he found that we had different last names, the male receptionist insisted that our rooms had to be on different floors.

Soon after that weekend I felt that I wanted to marry Mary. Mary was 25 and I was 30 so we were not rash teenagers. Mary's brother, Bill, was returning from California to take the examination for a professional engineer (P.E.) in January 1959, so Mary decided that would be the right time for the wedding. From my point of view, the Wisconsin winter was coming on and I did not relish digging my car out of the snow at night after visiting Mary. Thus the idea of marrying and moving in with Mary had a lot of appeal.

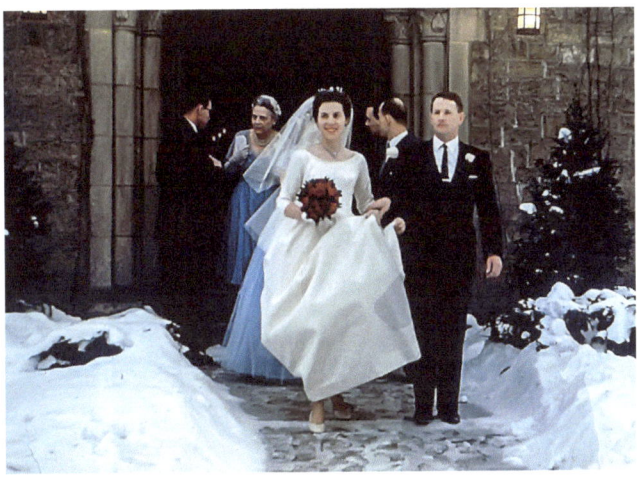

By the time of the wedding, Mary's parents had accepted me but her brother and many friends were skeptical. They thought that it was just another rushed American marriage which would end in divorce. In fact the marriage lasted until Mary's death over forty years later. The wedding took place at St. Francis House with Rev. Gerald White, who had introduced us, officiating. The date was January 24, 1959 a day on which the temperature rose above 0°F for the first time in 30 days!

As an example of the regard in which Mary was held, one of her clients offered the use of his family's cabin on the other side of Lake Mendota, in which we were able to spend the weekend. The cabin was magnificent, with a large walk-in stone fireplace and a huge picture window looking across the lake to the city of Madison. On the Sunday we hiked out onto the lake and watched the ice fishermen. Mary continued working with the furniture store and I worked to complete my doctorate. After the wedding, I persuaded Mary to sell her Thunderbird and we bought a 1957 Buick Convertible. During the summer of 1959 we took the honeymoon we were not able to take in January and drove up to Quebec City in Canada.

After my graduation in May 1960 we took a trip to Cornell University at Ithaca, NY, to see friends who were taking an advanced degree. We then drove on up to Boston, back through New York City and down to Washington, finally

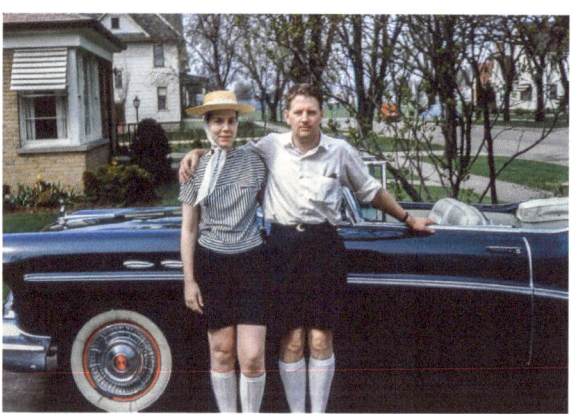

returning to Wisconsin via Kentucky, and Indiana. All the way on this trip we stayed with either Mary's friends or mine. The rest of that summer was spent getting ready for our trip to Australia where, as it would turn out, we would spend the first five years of married life.

LIFE IN AUSTRALIA...

Chapter 3

THE YEARS IN AUSTRALIA

Getting to Australia was complex. We were shipping many items including Mary's electric organ and a stove built at the plant where Mary's father worked. We also planned to take the Buick convertible. We sent the large wooden crates with our belongings by rail to San Francisco then drove the Buick west, where the car and the crates were placed on a ship. In San Francisco we enjoyed a last weekend together with Mary's brother. Then we boarded one of the first of the Pan Am 707 jets for the polar route to London. The jets had commenced operation only a short time before this. A fellow passenger on that flight was Alfred Hitchcock. Since the flight was over the Arctic, we were able to see a marvelous display of the Aurora Borealis.

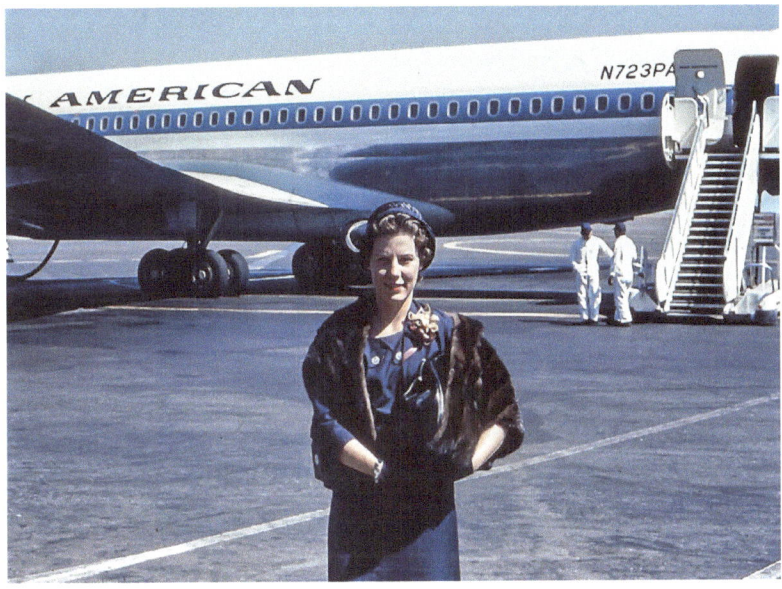

We spent a wonderful month in England and then met up with one of my university colleagues in Basel, Switzerland. This was a woman who had been a fellow graduate student in Madison. She accompanied us and acted as interpreter for the rest of our trip down through Italy to Naples where we boarded the P & O liner "Orcades" for the trip to Australia. This was fun with stops in the Suez Canal and Aden, on the coast of Arabia, and finally a day in Colombo in what was then Ceylon, now Sri Lanka.

Finally we arrived in Australia, and I realized I had been remiss in planning before I took my new bride Down Under. I did not have a job so we moved in with my parents, who had modified their home to provide a small apartment at the back. Such an arrangement was acceptable to Australians who were used to shortages of housing and other discomforts but it certainly placed a strain on a sophisticated American woman. In fact the cultural differences between the United States and Australia in the 1960s were much greater than either Mary or I had anticipated. One of Mary's first images was of sheep carcasses hanging on racks in the butchers' shops with saw dust on the floor. Rent control still hung over from the war and consequently apartments were almost unavailable. That first year put some strain on the marriage but Mary handled it well and made many firm friends both among Australians and Americans who were living in Sydney.

After several weeks, I interviewed with Sir Asher Joel who owned an advertising/public relations agency. He hired me as the director of his Motivational Research group. Asher Joel had been the Australian Naval Officer assigned to General MacArthur's staff during World War II. In that position he gained firsthand experience in the operation of public relations and became the first Australian member of the American Public Relations Association. In 1954 he was appointed as organizer of Queen Elizabeth's visit to Australia and since he did a great job he was knighted by the Queen. He was absolutely charming to Mary and we both maintained our friendship. Sir Asher visited America during the Bicentennial in 1976 and he and his wife came to our home for dinner. He died in 1999 a few months before Mary.

After I had a secure job we were able to spend weekends looking for an apartment. Eventually we found a new one bedroom apartment on the third floor of a block close to a commuter rail station. Mary took a part-time position as a decorator with a woman who had a small furniture business.

Sir Asher Joel, in addition to his position as head of the advertising agency was a member of the upper house of the state legislature and had a number of American connections. One of these was as a director of the American Club in Sydney. This was a major business Club with lavish premises in the city. There was also an American Society, more of an informal group of ex-patriot Americans and The American Women's Club. Sir Asher introduced Mary to the American Society and we became involved with their fun activities. Mary soon became very active in The American Women's Club and was eventually elected as their secretary. This was really quite an honor for Mary since other members were wives of senior executives of American corporations. The president was Ann Clark, the wife of the Australian Manager of Pan American Airways. Ann had been a U.S. Army nurse who was captured by the Japanese on Corregidor and had been highly decorated for the help she had given soldiers on the Bataan Death March.

With Sir Asher's connections and Mary's role in the American Women's Club we soon were participating in many social events. Mary and I were in the official party at the memorial service for General Douglas MacArthur. Then, since Sir Asher was ill at the time, we took his place at the formal dinner for Chief Justice Earl Warren when he visited Sydney and were seated at the head table.

Chapter 4

OUR FIRST DAUGHTER

After we had settled down in Sydney, Mary decided to consult a gynecologist for some minor problem. However, the gynecologist seemed to think she was concerned that, after three years of marriage, she was not pregnant. After a careful examination he indicated that Mary had Endometriosis, a condition in which some of the cells lining the uterus move up the fallopian tubes into the body cavity. It can cause severe pain and other complications if it is not treated. In the 1960s the only treatment was surgery.

The gynecologist with whom Mary had consulted was not bashful and indicated that he was a "world authority" on the disease and regularly went to San Francisco to consult at Stanford University concerning Endometriosis. He went on to say that 90% of the women on whom he had operated had conceived within the year. We would have to make up our minds quickly if we wanted him to perform the operation as he was leaving for San Francisco within two months, then he would go on to South America and finally to a major conference in Moscow. After much debate, Mary elected to have the operation, which she got through with a scar all the way down from her navel.

The Doctor with a rather cavalier attitude said "the right ovary was so encased in cells that I just took it out". This may or may not have been significant in her later development of Alzheimer's disease. It is now known that insufficient estrogen is possibly a risk factor in the occurrence of Alzheimer's disease. It can be argued that one ovary can produce as much estrogen as is needed, but at menopause one ovary may stop producing estrogen sooner than might occur with two functioning ovaries. The gynecologist was correct on one thing. Mary became pregnant within about six months of the operation.

Shortly after the operation, we were out for a drive on a cold foggy afternoon and we drove down a road that had just been opened in one of the northern suburbs of Sydney. This was a new land development and there, in the fog, was the original home which had occupied the property before its subdivision. It was a Cape-Cod style house in white brick with a slate roof and two dormer windows in the front. Mary was delighted with it and we eventually bought the house.

Mary applied her decorating talents and I worked on the landscaping. As further evidence of Mary's decorating ability, the restored home was featured in the October 1964 issue of Australian House and Garden Magazine. The kitchen was completely re-built and we installed the Monarch stove we had brought from Wisconsin. After lots of work everything was ready by the time the baby was due. In fact Mary was still wallpapering when her water broke at about 11 p.m.

I called the doctor and was told to get Mary to the hospital as soon as possible. We arrived about 1 am. Since there had been no preparation for natural childbirth and there was no thought of me being present at the birth I went home and on to work at the regular time. About 2 p.m. I received a phone call informing me that we had a daughter. She was named Elizabeth Claire, and was born on May 15, 1963.

Elizabeth was healthy and happy and developed quickly. In September 1963 Mary's mother and father came to Australia to see the new granddaughter. While they were with us we took them on a trip in our station wagon out into western part of the state of New South Wales and on to Australia's capital city, Canberra.

For the four years after returning to Australia, I had attempted, without success, to interest Australian Universities in establishing a department of Agricultural Extension. In the early 1960s Rachael Carson wrote the book *Silent Spring*. As a result of that book the U.S. Congress appropriated money to study the way in which pesticides are used. The U.S. Department of Agriculture received some of that special funding and established a research project to develop a national plan for training all groups of people in the correct use of pesticides. I was asked to direct that project and so our small family decided to return to the United States in April of 1965. Mary had really settled into life in Australia and was not especially anxious to go through the problems of another move. But we put the house on the market and packed our things.

Then about three weeks prior to departure she was infected with a serious case of influenza and her temperature rose to 104°F. The infection developed into cystitis (a urinary infection). A few days before our actual departure, Mary needed to pay one last visit to her gynecologist in Sydney. As usual, Mary took the commuter train to the city - a trip of about 20 minutes. Commuter trains did not have toilet facilities and during the trip Mary needed to urinate. In panic she left the train at its first stop before her city destination and rushed to a rest room at that station. After several more stops at toilets she eventually saw the doctor and he prescribed an anti-biotic which soon cleared the cystitis.

However the panic of needing to urinate when no toilet facilities were available remained with Mary for at least three years. Such panic attacks can be a manifestation of clinical depression and Mary may have been suffering from depression but she did not show other symptoms. I mention this because there is sometimes confusion between early signs of Alzheimer's disease and depression.

In retrospect, I wonder if the influenza and the resulting urinary tract infection may well have been the cause that led to development of Alzheimer's disease many years later. Later in this book there is a discussion of a new theory that Alzheimer's disease may result from infection with the bacteria *Clostridium pneumoniae*.

We left Sydney as planned, on QANTAS airlines, and my parents were devastated as they watched us walk out to the gangway (the days before Jet ways) with little Elizabeth trotting between us.

LIFE IN AMERICA...

CHAPTER 5

IN FORT COLLINS

The project which I was to direct for the U.S. Department of Agriculture was based at Colorado State University so we planned to go directly to Fort Collins, Colorado. Mary had recovered somewhat from the cystitis infection which had resulted from her bout with influenza but it apparently left a residual problem. Major household items which we wanted in America were packed in large boxes and picked up for sea shipment by a forwarding company. All other items we owned were sold or given away.

Our house had been on the market for a month or more but had not sold by the time we had to leave for America so reluctantly we were forced to leave it in the hands of a realtor. Fortunately he was able to close a sale within 6 weeks of our departure. Our sale price was £10,000 - at that time (1965) roughly equivalent to $18,000.

Before leaving Australia we had arranged to rent a furnished apartment until we could move into a home which we planned to buy. The apartment was ready for us, so the next day we went house hunting. Very quickly we found a ranch style house on the edge of town and signed a contract. Almost immediately I had to travel to Washington, DC to meet with my supervisor in the head office of the U.S. Department of Agriculture. There was snow on the ground in Ft. Collins when I left but it was beautiful spring weather in Washington with the cherry trees out and the azaleas blooming. Mary fared quite well in the apartment while I was away for about ten days.

Soon after my return to Ft. Collins we moved into the home we had purchased. We settled into a regular routine with me driving about half a mile to my office on the campus of the university and Mary staying home with Elizabeth. We shopped together after I returned home from work and members of the faculty and their wives took us into their social groups. Mary was soon asked to join the American Society of University Women (AAUW).

Panic attacks, which Mary had first experienced in Australia, came on again after our arrival in Fort Collins. The problem was intermittent and not particularly serious. On one occasion, Mary and I were shopping in a supermarket; Mary appeared to have the urge to urinate and insisted on leaving immediately. We left the grocery cart where it was and departed quickly. A few weeks later we were invited to a reception for new faculty at the home of the president of Colorado State University. Approximately 15 minutes after arrival Mary indicated that she had to urinate, I suggested that we look for the lady's room. However, Mary insisted that we go home immediately. We did so and approximately two hours later, I noticed that Mary had not gone to the toilet since our return. It was obvious that the problem was mental. On reflection we recalled that Mary's father had a somewhat similar problem with urinary frequency when away from home.

Again I wondered if a mental cause for urinary frequency may be related to the onset of Alzheimer's disease. After the first few months in Ft. Collins Mary seemed to get over the panic attacks.

From my point of view, the two years in Fort Collins were probably two of the best years of my life. On the other hand Mary always felt that Fort Collins was culturally isolated. Every other month I went for briefings at the U.S. Department of Agriculture headquarters in Washington. Mary stayed home with Elizabeth and only went out to meetings of AAUW. In our second year in Fort Collins, Mary decided to send Elizabeth to Montessori School and then she had more time to meet with faculty wives and become involved in many other activities.

On a number of occasions I had to visit agricultural extension services in surrounding states. On those occasions I was able to take Mary and Elizabeth with me. We also were able to take long weekends and vacation time to visit many of the tourist sites of the western U.S.A. These trips included locations such as Yellowstone Park, Mesa Verde Indian ruins, and the narrow gauge railroad from Durango to Silverton. One particularly nice thing about Fort Collins was that, at lunch time on a Sunday afternoon we could decide that it would be nice to go to the mountains and within two hours we could be in the snow at 12,000 feet in Rocky Mountain National Park. Besides the entertainment resources of Denver which were only about an hour and a half away, there was the famous opera house at Central City.

Fort Collins is an extremely pleasant city. While it is at about 6,000 feet elevation it is certainly not in the mountains. The city is on the western edge of the high plains and is quite flat and treeless except for plantings on the streets and people's gardens. The foothills of the Rocky Mountains start about 10 miles west of the city, and beyond them one enters several canyons, the most significant of which is the Cache La Poudre Canyon, so named because it was where French fur trappers kept their store of gunpowder.

Proceeding up those canyons takes one into the heavily forested main mountains of the Rockies and one is soon at 10 to 11,000 feet. Interstate highway I-25 runs from Fort Collins into Denver and when we lived there it was quite new and provided us with a very fast way to Denver.

Colorado State University has a lot going for it but when I was doing some research work with a professor at Iowa State University I found that he owned land in the mountains nearby. I asked him why, when he owned land near Fort Collins, he did not take a faculty appointment at CSU. His answer was, "They trade salary for scenery."

For the two Christmas seasons that we lived in Fort Collins, we drove the 1,000 miles back to Beaver Dam, to celebrate the holidays with Mary's parents. These were great trips and apart from the usual snow in Wisconsin, we only encountered light snow throughout the trips and the roads were not closed.

In the summer of 1966 my mother and father visited us in Fort Collins. My father was delighted to get to see Fort Collins because the library at CSU had purchased a copy of a book he had written many years before. The weather was wonderful and I took a number of vacation days.

It was after a trip to Yellowstone National Park when we discovered that our small family was growing. Mary was pregnant again!

Our second child Margaret was born in the Poudre Valley Hospital in Fort Collins on May 5, 1967. During the summer of 1967 the Pesticide project on which I was working came to an end. After a lot of investigation I accepted a position as a Chief of Information at the Centers for Disease Control (CDC), U.S. Public Health Service which was located in Atlanta.

We were moving again…

CHAPTER 6

IN ATLANTA

By Labor Day 1967 our house in Fort Collins was sold, we packed a large U-Haul trailer and set off in the station wagon for Atlanta. Soon after arrival we purchased a nice home in Chamblee, a north eastern suburb. Now, Atlanta in the mid 1960s was a very different place from the present city. The population was predominately born there and closely attached to family - Uncles, Aunts, cousins etc. Those from outside were not well accepted even though the locals were always saying "we are so friendly", "we will have to get together sometime".

In fact, several months after we arrived, I was working in the yard when our immediate next door neighbor walked over and said "Hi, my name's Fred, we will have to get together some time." In the 10 months we spent in Atlanta that was the only time we ever saw Fred. At that time, I held a GS 14 grade in the U.S. Civil Service, a relatively high level. However we were never invited to visit in anyone else's home. This was in marked contrast with all other cities where we had lived. In all those cases Mary made friends quickly and we were always going out to friends' homes for dinner or inviting them to our home. Mary was an excellent cook and the dinners were events which friends still recall when I meet them.

Difficult as Atlanta was for me, it was a disaster for Mary. The locals were still fighting General Sherman, who, as you know was from Wisconsin. Mary was considered as a "dammed Yankee". She had no friends. In fact she said that the only people she was ever able to talk with were the check-out girls at the super market. We joined the local Episcopal Church but Mary was never invited to participate in any activities. After six months she enrolled Elizabeth in the local Montessori school and was able to work out a car pool arrangement with a neighbor. Wishing to be friendly, she asked the woman if she and her husband would care to come to our home for drinks on the following Sunday afternoon. The woman said "That's nice but Bill always watches the game on TV"! Not that they had <u>tickets</u> to the game.

One of the crowning blows for Mary came at Christmas time. As had been our custom in Wisconsin and Australia, she decided to have a Christmas party. Invitations were sent to 36 people. Apologies were received from three people and Mary prepared food for 33. When, on the appointed day, only two couples and one single man showed up, Mary was devastated.

In June of 1968 I was approached by a research company, Pennsylvania Research Associates. After an interview they made me an offer which was part time with them and part time directing a project that the National Library of Medicine had contracted with the University of Pennsylvania. Because of our dislike of Atlanta I accepted the offer and we moved, once again, this time to Philadelphia. A few weeks before departure Mary and I visited Philadelphia and purchased a new house on the "Main Line".

CHAPTER 7

IN PHILADELPHIA

We arrived in Philadelphia in mid July and I started right in to work. By this time we had two cars, a new Pontiac station wagon and a small MG. I was able to drive the small car to the railroad and then take a commuter train to the city. This left Mary with the station wagon and plenty of time to look after the two girls. In the fall of 1968 Elizabeth was enrolled in the local grade school which was a bus ride of almost 10 miles from our home. Our family settled in to life in Philadelphia very quickly. We joined the Episcopal Church which was within easy walking distance of our home. The Church immediately provided us with a wide circle of friends.

While we were by no means fundamentalists, the local Episcopal Church, St. David's, did form a basis for much of our social contacts. St. David's was built by Welsh settlers in 1715. In fact the church communion service had been given by Queen Anne. The old original church holds only about 100 people. This church was filled to overflowing for Mary's funeral some 31 years later. A chapel accommodating about 500 was built in 1955. The church membership when we arrived was in the order of 3,000.

After approximately two years in Philadelphia, Mary joined with two other women and organized a church supper club. Each month the group met in the home of one of the members. The host family provided the entrée and the other members bring salads, vegetables and desserts which are shared. The supper club group at St. David's grew so that eventually there were three divisions each of about 30 families. As our first daughter, Elizabeth progressed to fourth grade, Mary decided to help out by becoming a Sunday school teacher.

The next church activity for Mary was her election as president of the Episcopal Church Women at St. David's. She assumed this position in 1975. In 1978 she was sent as a Pennsylvania delegate to the convention of the Episcopal Church which was held in New Orleans. I also participated in the life of the church and was elected to the vestry of St. David's. In an Episcopal church the vestry is the local governing body of lay members of the congregation of each parish. Eventually I became the Junior Warden - the second lay person in the congregation.

We went to Philadelphia so that I could take up employment at Pennsylvania Research Associates and the University of Pennsylvania. By the end of 1969 I decided to form my own company, Educational Communications Inc.(ECI). Our purpose was to produce training programs for use by Fortune 500 companies to train their employees in regional locations all over the world. When our company was incorporated, Mary became the legal Secretary/Treasurer. At first I was the only employee and I continued on a part-time basis to direct the project at the University of Pennsylvania. As the work in the company expanded and more people were employed, Mary began to take an active part in all activities. She was primarily responsible for payroll and bookkeeping. She also participated with me in interviewing all new employees.

One of the clients of ECI was the automobile manufacturer, British Leyland (at that time maker of MGs, Triumphs, and Jaguars). In 1975 ECI contracted to develop audiovisual programs and manuals to train the mechanics at the Leyland dealers throughout America on the intricacies of particular systems, such as air conditioning, brakes, etc. These programs were so appreciated by dealers in the United States that the parent company in England asked me to visit them and plan to produce similar programs for British Leyland on a world-wide basis. We therefore formed another company, Service Training Limited, in England. Mary was also appointed as a legal director of the English company.

This arrangement enabled me to visit England every three months. Mary accompanied me approximately every second trip. There was a lot of work to be done while in England, but we were also able to spend the weekends traveling around Britain. Service Training Limited grew and soon we were developing the world-wide training materials for Rolls Royce Cars and then others such as BMW, and Ford (UK).

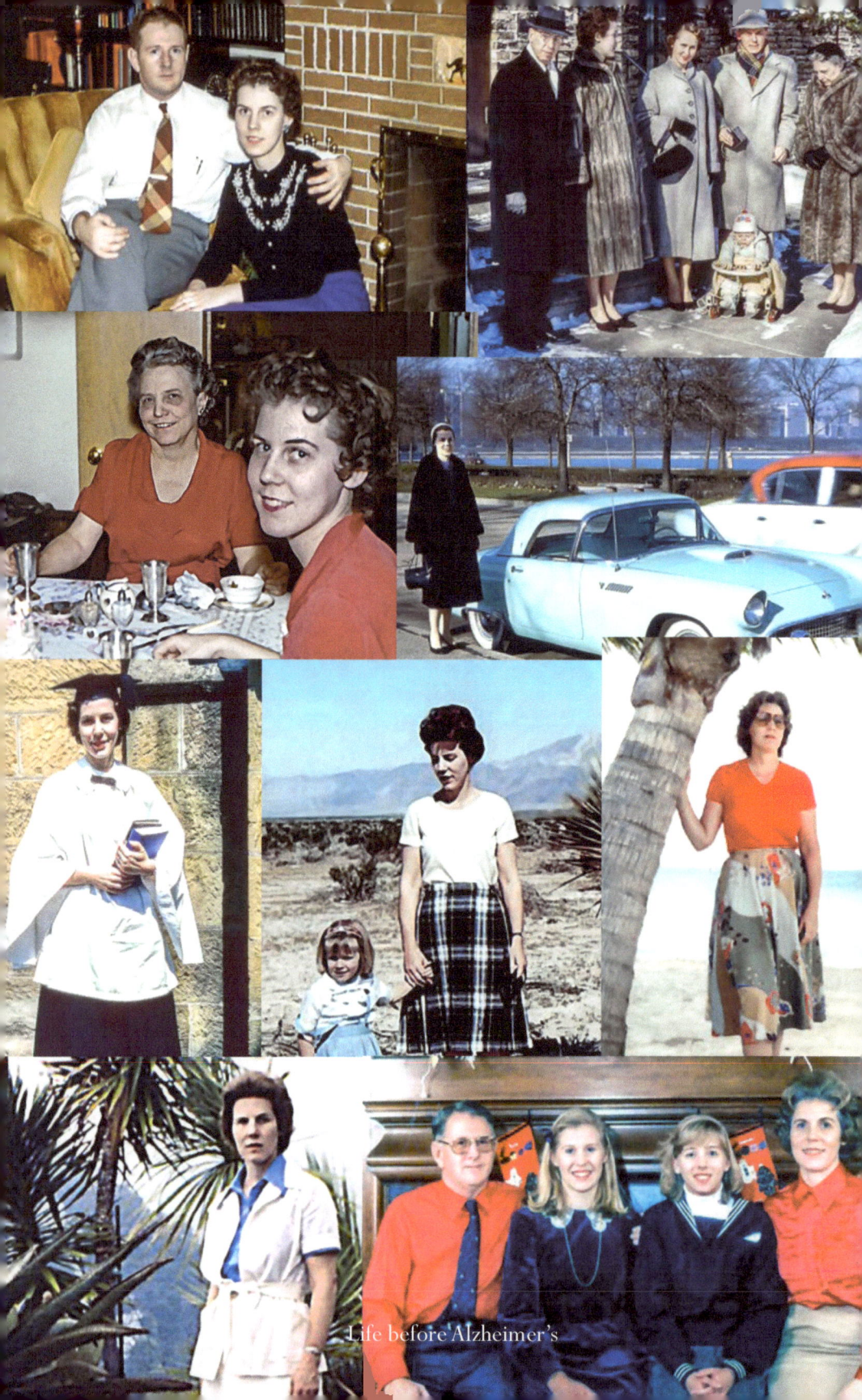

Life before Alzheimer's

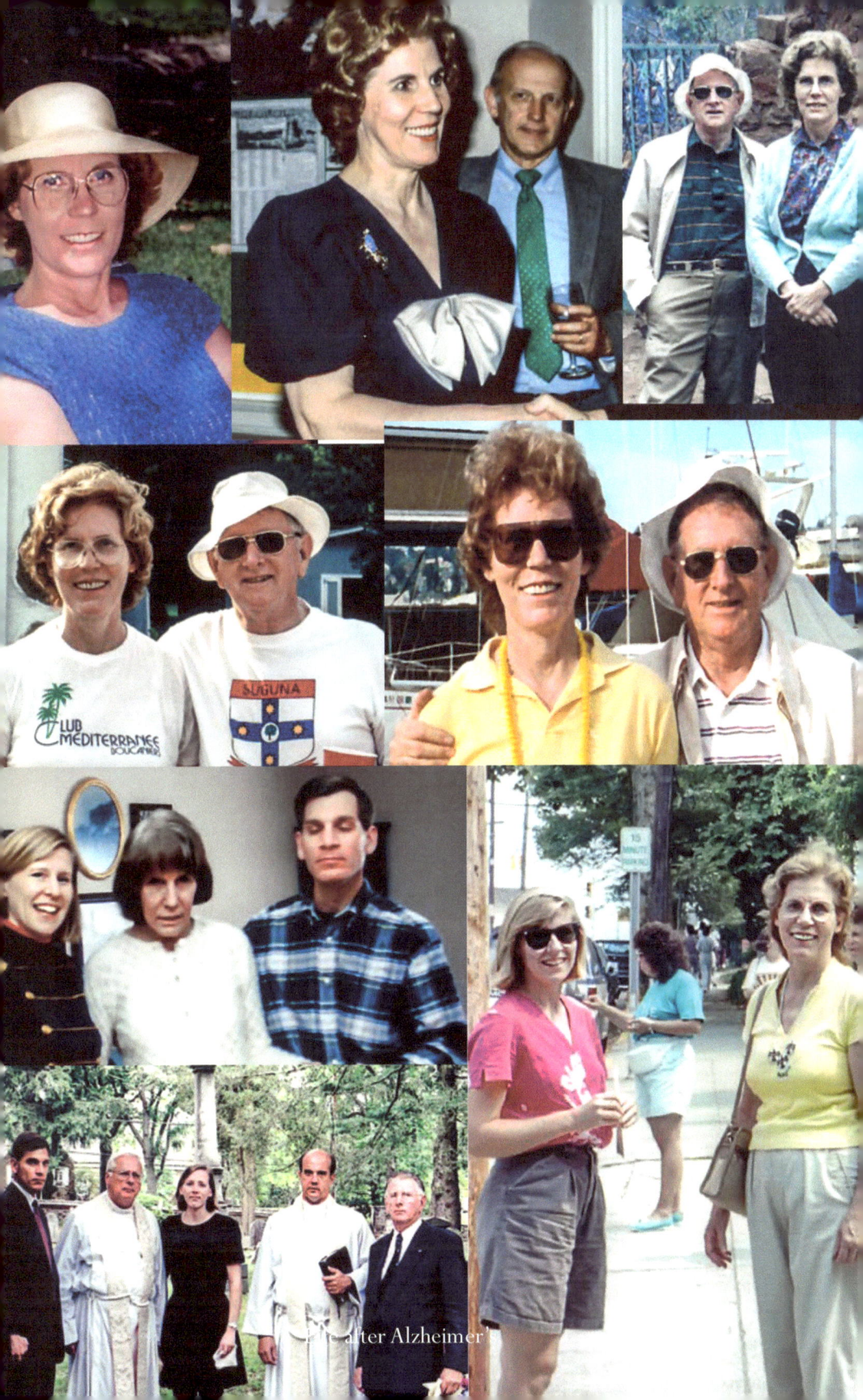

Life after Alzheimer's

LIFE UNRAVELS...

CHAPTER 8

THE FIRST INKLING OF TROUBLE

We were living a relatively full life with extensive travel that Mary enjoyed immensely. That life was about to change.

In 1980 Mary was asked if she would run for president of the local chapter of the American Association of University Women (AAUW). Surprisingly she refused this. In considering this in retrospect, it is possible that Mary was sensing a problem and felt she could not do justice to the position.

There were also problems at our company. Mary learned to use a word processor in the days prior to personal computers. In spite of her typing ability, she experienced a lot of difficulty remembering what she needed to do to save material to a floppy disk or to print it out.

Then, one Friday evening in 1984 I arrived home just as our younger daughter Margaret, who was a junior in high school at that time, was leaving in her car. Margaret told me that she was going to dinner with her boy friend. I said, "Great, have a good time". Mary and I then had dinner and spent the evening together. About 11 p.m. Margaret was not home and so Mary and I talked about what might have happened. Mary expressed surprise that Margaret had not returned by that time. Not wishing to be the worrying parent, I decided to sleep on it. Then, as Margaret was not home when we awoke on Saturday morning, I was very worried and shared my worry with Mary. She also expressed amazement.

By noon, as I was about to phone the family of Margaret's boyfriend, she walked in. Understandably I was very annoyed with her for staying the night with her boyfriend. Margaret's response was, "oh Daddy, as I was leaving I told Mommy that, after dinner, I was going to spend the night with Molly so we could do some homework assignments". Mary's response was that she did not remember that.

At the time Margaret and I did not know it but, this was the first clear indication of Alzheimer's. Normal people all forget things, such as, they fail to do something or they fail to recall something. When reminded of what was missed they will say, "Oh, I forgot I had to do that, or oh, yes I must have forgotten". What is different with the Alzheimer's sufferer is that they cannot recall something which they were told only the day before or often only a few hours before. At that stage Mary was not failing to remember other things, such as what day it was, or who "Molly" was.

The problem Mary had at that stage was not so much "loss of memory" as the fact that certain information was never stored into memory. The next occurrence was several months later. The vice president of Educational Communications came to me and said "I am worried about Mary, I asked her to attend to a matter relating to one of the employees and she agreed to do it. Now only a few days later, when it was not attended to, I asked her about it and she does not recall that we had discussed it."

In 1986, I brought a partner into the business. After a few months he suggested that it was better not to have the wife of the president as an employee and so Mary resigned.

Several friends then offered Mary jobs. One was with an insurance company and would have involved some typing. Mary looked at these offers and turned them all down. In retrospect it must have been apparent to her that she would not be able to perform. Also in 1986 we decided that Mary should consult our local general practitioner. He ordered tests for endocrine conditions, blood work, etc. He then declared to me that if all his patients were as healthy as Mary he would be out of business. This condition, where the sufferer is in good health, apart from the deterioration in mental capacity, seems to be a characteristic of Alzheimer's disease. Many sufferers are extremely fit in all other respects.

Mary's doctor suggested that she might be suffering from depression and referred her to a psychologist. She had a number of sessions with that person. In interviews she expressed the view that the family had moved location too frequently but there was little else that came out. At this stage none of the doctors or the psychologist suggested dementia or Alzheimer's. In those years the condition was not in the public arena.

Early in 1987 we decided that the big old house, in which we had lived for 12 years, should be sold. Elizabeth was through college and Margaret was a junior in college. Obviously a smaller house would be more suitable. We rented a house in a nearby development while we looked for a new home. One of our problems in that search was what we could do with all the possessions we had acquired and which fitted nicely into the big house? I think that having to dispose of things is a factor that is particularly traumatic for a person starting to experience Alzheimer's disease and therefore has undue influence on family decisions that should be made at that time.

After much searching, we decided to build the house that we had always wanted, and as Margaret was completing a degree in architecture from Rhode Island School of Design she prepared the basic designs. At this time Mary was functioning quite well and actively participating in all the decisions concerning the house.

In the mid 1980s I was serving as president of the Philadelphia Chapter of the Wisconsin Alumni Association. One evening in the spring of 1988 Mary and I attended a dinner with members of the Alumni Association, and seated at our table was Dr. Justin Parr a physician who was serving as a research associate at the University of Pennsylvania. As we were leaving the dinner, Dr. Parr took me aside and said, "I think Mary may be suffering from Alzheimer's disease." He went on to say that the Department of Gerontology at the University of Pennsylvania had a project to investigate the diagnosis of Alzheimer's and he would be pleased to get Mary into the program.

With some effort, I managed to persuade Mary to participate in the program. She was admitted to the Hospital of the University of Pennsylvania (HUP) on July 26, 1988 for two days of tests. These included total blood work-up, Cat scans, MRI, and a battery of psychological tests, such as drawings, counting backwards from one hundred by intervals of seven, etc. Also Mary was given one of the earliest PET scans used for the diagnosis of Alzheimer's disease. This is Positron Emission Tomography, a test that evaluates the chemical activity in different parts of the brain. One of the reasons for admission to the hospital was that because of the very high cost of the PET scan machines they schedule them 24 hours per day and Mary was tested in the early hours of the morning. Mary was discharged from HUP on July 28, 1988.

Dr. Chawluk, who was directing this research program at HUP asked Elizabeth and me to call at the hospital for a review of Mary's test results. At that time Dr. Chawluk informed us that his diagnosis was probably Alzheimer's disease. He showed us the PET scans of Mary's brain and pointed out the areas of diminished activity.

After Elizabeth and I had received the news of Mary's condition we returned home and told her about it. It is difficult to say whether she fully understood the implications but this was one of the few times she had been known to cry about her own condition.

CHAPTER 9

DIAGNOSTIC RESULTS

These are the details of Mary's discharge summary, prepared by Dara Jamieson, M.D. an associate in the Alzheimer's disease research center at HUP.

PHYSICAL EXAMINATION

Mary's blood pressure was 138/80, pulse was 80 and regular; her HEENT exam was unremarkable; lungs clear; cardiac exam was normal S1, S2; abdominal exam showed normal active bowel sounds; non-tender abdomen; pulses were intact in her extremities.

NEUROLOGICAL EXAMINATION

On neurological examination she was alert and cooperative and would respond to questioning, however, there was no spontaneous speech and she rarely volunteered information. Her mini mental status examination score was 23. She showed difficulty with orientation, and she was unable to remember three objects after an interval of five minutes.

LABORATORY DATA

On admission she revealed normal electrolytes. Liver function tests were normal. Hemoglobin was 14.8; white count was 7.2, with normal differential. Triglycerides were 468 and cholesterol was 187. UA was unremarkable. PT was slightly prolonged at 14.8 while the normal range is 10-13. Her PTT was normal at 27. EKG showed normal sinus rhythm with prolonged QT and right atrial enlargement. Chest x-ray was normal. MRI of the brain showed normal brain parenchyma with the exception of several small high signal intensities in the right frontal white matter. These were interpreted as nonspecific findings.

The ventricles were of normal size but the sulci were prominent bilaterally. Her ischemia score for dementia was 0 indicating probable Alzheimer's disease. Her dementia scale was 8. This would indicate mild to moderate impairment of activities of daily living. Her vascular risk factor score was low at 2. Carotid real-time ultrasonography was normal. EEG was read as mildly abnormal because of focal slowing and disorganization of background activity over the left cerebral hemisphere. No epileptiform activity was observed. Mary was unable to tolerate a regional cerebral blood flow scan. Her PET scan showed mild posterior parietal and occipital association areas of hypometabolism.

NEURO-PSYCHOLOGIC TESTING

Neuro-psychologic testing showed that Mary had an average fund of information, visual special skills and perceptual speed with above average vocabulary. Conceptual flexibility was moderately impaired. She had difficulties with slow performance. Digit span was average, forward and reverse. Memory and learning tasks were severely impaired. Marked difficulty with immediate and delayed verbal memory as well as with verbal list learning was evident. Her visual memory, both immediate and delayed, was also severely impaired. Her language testing with fluency and sentence comprehension and repetition was normal to low normal. Her depression scale was in the mild range for depression. The conclusion was that there had been a decline in intellectual functioning from her premorbid level. Most striking was the degree of memory impairment with little information and then coded and then no recall following a 30 minute delay. This was considered to be compatible with Alzheimer's disease.

In summary it shows that Mary was in quite good physical condition with no major medical problems other than moderate to severe reduction in brain functioning.

Another point to remember is that through 2001 there was no precise way to diagnose Alzheimer's disease until the brain is examined following death. The above medical report shows the extensive testing which can lead to a presumption of Alzheimer's disease.

It should be emphasized that in the early stages of Alzheimer's disease the patient has not so much <u>lost</u> memory but is experiencing difficulty in processing, storing and interpreting new information.

Chapter 10

CAR AND DRIVER

After the diagnosis, things returned to normal or as near normal as they could be. Construction commenced on the house. Mary was active in watching over the construction and was very helpful with advice and suggestions. She continued to drive her car and meet with friends. Virtually no one except our closest friends suspected or knew of Mary's condition.

About a month after the meeting at which Dr. Chawluk had informed me of the diagnosis, he scheduled a follow-up visit. At that visit he prescribed Prozac, as he thought she was likely to exhibit depression, and he advised that she should take lecithin. Dr. Chawluk explained that, as Alzheimer's disease causes a breakdown in nerve cells and blocks neuro-transmission there was a need to try to improve the transmission of impulses between the nerve cells which were still functioning. Remember this was 1988 and there were not any specific products for treatment of Alzheimer's disease.

Transmission of impulses between nerves is assisted by a chemical, acetylcholine, and Dr. Chawluk suggested that there appears to be a deficiency of this chemical in the Alzheimer's patient. Lecithin, manufactured from soy beans, is a common name for phosphatidylcholines which are components of cell membranes. It has been suggested that lecithin may assist in the synthesis of acetylcholine.

Because there are several varieties of lecithin some with saturated fatty acids, some with unsaturated fatty acids, and others with a mixture of saturated and unsaturated fatty acids, Dr. Chawluk recommended that I should get pure medical lecithin directly from the American Lecithin Company. It is a white, or slightly cream, waxy powder which Mary took mixed with cereal.

One interesting fact was that Mary took a strong dislike both to Dr. Chawluk and to Dr. Parr. There was no apparent reason for this. Dr. Parr certainly had never examined her and Dr. Chawluk probably had not examined her. Neither doctor had conversed with her to any extent. It is possible that she saw them as being privy to her secret, or in some way she may have subconsciously blamed them for her condition.

As we will see, at a later stage of her disease she continually insisted that there was nothing wrong with her. She was always saying that I was the one who was sick and needed to see a doctor. It is possible that subconsciously she feared that I might be sick and therefore might not be able to care for her.

In May 1989 the house was completed. We moved in and immediately drove to Providence, Rhode Island to attend the graduation of our daughter Margaret. Mary was able to participate and had an almost normal time on that trip. On returning to Malvern there were all the things that had to be done to get the new house in order. Margaret took a job with an architectural firm in Philadelphia and came to live in her room in the new house. Elizabeth also occupied her room as she was working as a pilot for Du Pont, based in Wilmington, Delaware and was able to commute.

During the day, while I was at work, Mary was by herself, but found plenty to do working on the house and garden. She still drove her car to the supermarket and to have her hair done. We attended our normal social gatherings and as I mentioned above almost no one knew that there was anything wrong with Mary. In October, 1989 we held a big house-warming party. Mary sent the invitations and participated in the entertainment.

At this time Mary was losing interest in reading in any meaningful way. It was apparent that, because she had forgotten what she had read on earlier pages, the text was failing to make sense. Through 1992 she was able to read sentences and through 1994 she could still read single words. Gradually her writing deteriorated, but she was still able to sign her name in a meaningful way through the end of 1993.

Had there not been a relatively definitive diagnosis of Alzheimer's disease in 1988 and considering Mary's age it is probable that a lot of her symptoms would have been unrecognized at least until 1992. I mention this because it is often said that people with Alzheimer's disease may die within 5 years of diagnosis. It is more probable that the disease is present for a longer period but goes unrecognized until it is well advanced. In fact, while we had the diagnosis in July 1988 it is most probable that Mary was experiencing some of the effects of Alzheimer's as early as 1980. Our daughter Margaret insists that she felt her mother was not functioning properly long before Elizabeth and I first noticed it.

Very shortly after Dr. Chawluk had diagnosed Mary as suffering from Alzheimer's disease, he left the Hospital of the University of Pennsylvania. Mary then came under the care of a woman, Dr. Dara Jamieson, with whom she had several visits at the hospital. In most cases the doctor asked Mary simple questions such as what day it was and where they were. She usually had little trouble with these questions. In fact at that time Mary was still functioning relatively well. It was interesting that while Mary had taken a strong dislike to Drs. Chawluk and Parr, and that in the past she had not liked female doctors, she seemed to get on quite well with Dr. Jamieson.

As there was no approved drug for the treatment of Alzheimer's disease there seemed to be little benefit to be gained from visiting a physician. Mary had no obvious physical sickness and little was to be gained by continuing to talk with a doctor. Because Dr. Chawluk had prescribed "Prozac" it was necessary to continue to have prescriptions written. Mary's primary care physician was reluctant to write these prescriptions and therefore recommended that she consult a psychiatrist. On two occasions Mary visited a local psychiatrist. All he did was talk with her and little seemed to be accomplished. Once again Mary took a strong dislike to this doctor and it certainly was not worth the aggravation of persuading her to continue to visit him.

It is important to stress that Alzheimer's disease is a neurological disease and not a psychiatric disease. It is due to an anatomical deterioration in the brain cells and not due to an alteration in the brain chemistry. I believe that psychiatrists can do little to improve the condition of the Alzheimer's patient. Neurologists can possibly give some indication as to what parts of the brain are deteriorating and can now prescribe drugs (such as Cognex) which may slow the deterioration.

As mentioned, Mary continued to drive her car. Both our daughters and I frequently drove with her and observed her performance. She handled the car well and reacted appropriately. During 1992 the family changed their dentist. On several occasions I went with Mary to the new dentist who was in Gladwyne, a suburb located approximately half way between our home in Malvern and downtown Philadelphia. Then Mary elected to visit the dentist several times on her own. One day when Mary had gone to visit the dentist, I received a phone call from her and learned that she was somewhere in the city. She had become lost and driven past the dentist's office and continued into Philadelphia. Fortunately I was able to instruct her as to how to get back on the expressway and return home. It was then apparent that Mary was unable to drive anywhere that was unfamiliar to her, but we continued to let her drive to the local supermarket.

In 1989 Dr. Jamieson moved from the Hospital of the University of Pennsylvania to Temple University School of Medicine and notified us of her new location. We chose not to continue to visit her in the new location. However, she then notified us that Temple University had established a center in King of Prussia which was near our company office, so in August, 1992 we scheduled an appointment at the center. Dr. Jamieson gave Mary a limited physical exam then asked Mary to put back the items of clothing she had removed and left the room. On returning the doctor found that Mary had completely undressed. On further discussion the doctor found that Mary had driven herself to the appointment even though I had followed in another car. Dr. Jamieson was horrified. She pointed out that under no circumstances should Mary be driving. She went on to point out that should there be a major accident, she as the attending physician, could be in trouble for failing to direct that the patient must NOT drive.

Following this session with Dr. Jamieson, we sold Mary's car. At the time my business was deteriorating and it was explained to Mary that we had to sell the car to provide money. Most relatives permit the patient to continue driving a car for far too long.

Dr. Peter Lipski, a geriatric medicine specialist, speaking at the International Association of Gerontology Conference held in Australia in August 1997 reported on a study which showed that, in Australia, some 80,000 persons with dementia are still driving their cars. On a comparison of the total population of Australia and the U.S.A. that would equate to 5 million demented Americans who are still driving. In the study, Dr. Lipski reported that persons who could not give their address or who did not know the time or the day were among those still driving.

It is probable that in August of 1992 Mary may not have been able to give her address nor say what day it was. Because of her former high level of intelligence, she was able to cover many situations. Thus, unless a person asked a direct question, she was able to evade disclosing that she was demented. Frequently, when at a party, someone would ask where her daughters were living. She would always say "I don't remember" and turn to me and say "Where is Margaret living now?" I would answer for her. Thus the episode would pass away and the questioner would probably not realize Mary had any problem.

Permitting Alzheimer's patients to continue driving is not only a serious danger to the patient but also a danger to other drivers. Inquiries reveal that the police are not able to take away driving privileges until an accident or major traffic infringement has occurred. Relatives are reluctant to force the patient to give up driving. Sons or daughters say "mom only drives to church or to the supermarket and we cannot take away her independence". It must therefore be physicians who should insist that the patient stops driving as soon as Alzheimer's disease is diagnosed.

For several years following the loss of her car, Mary claimed that she was having problems because her car had been taken away and she was unable to get about. Her car, and the independence it provided, was a very important factor for her. This loss of the car caused a lot of moderately violent arguments between us. The loss of driving privileges also seems to be a major concern for most Alzheimer's sufferers. When Mary was in the nursing home and I was sitting with her during meals I frequently heard conversation between the other residents relating that their cars had been "stolen".

CHAPTER 11

TRAVELING TOGETHER

Most couples look forward to traveling together in their years of retirement but for us it was obvious that this was not to be. I decided to continue taking as many trips as possible during the years in which Mary was still able to function in a more or less normal manner.

We had traveled very effectively together in England during the years when we owned the company there. In February 1986 after a hard winter we decided to take one of the short special vacations to the Bahamas. This was during the time of the Chernobyl atomic accident in Russia, the main item on the news, but Mary did not seem to understand it. Compared with earlier travel she was somewhat "out of it" during this trip to the Bahamas even though at that time it was not known that she was suffering from Alzheimer's Disease.

The first major trip after the diagnosis of Alzheimer's disease was a trip to Australia. Elizabeth and I were jointly presenting a paper at the 41st International Air Safety Conference held in Sydney during December 1988. That trip went well and Mary enjoyed meeting all her former friends. She recognized them and was able to continue a normal relationship with them. Only several very close friends were told of Mary's condition and they could not understand it because as they said, "she seemed so normal."

The Canadian Pacific Railroad had always had a strong appeal to both of us. In fact Mary had traveled back from her brother's wedding in Oregon on the Canadian Pacific Railroad and as a boy in Australia I had watched many beautiful travelogues produced by the Canadian Pacific Railroad. In 1990 I found that regular passenger trains had stopped running across Canada, however a small company was running special weekly tourist trains from Vancouver to Calgary. In September 1990 we took that trip. Since Mary's brother Bill lives in Seattle, we flew there and Bill and his wife drove us to Vancouver to catch the train to Banff. Everything considered that was a very pleasant vacation but I had to take much more care of Mary. She was unable to initiate anything on her own.

Ever since the war years when Churchill had gone to Marrakesh following the Casablanca conference, I had wanted to visit Morocco. In the winter of 1990-91 I made reservations for us to go to the Club Med resort in Marrakesh. However, in February 1991 as the time to depart arrived, the Gulf War broke out. Americans were then strongly advised not to visit a Muslm country. Because we could not get a refund we transferred to the Club Med resort at Playa Blanco in Mexico.

Everything considered that vacation at Club Med in Mexico also went well. Again we encountered another of those strange coincidences. After checking in to our cabin in the resort I found that one of my long-term employees and his wife were in the cabin next to us. The only problem we had on that trip concerned one of the activities, archery. Mary had been an active member of the Archery Club at the University of Wisconsin, so we both signed up.

The instructor was a Frenchman. He became very frustrated that Mary was unable to correctly handle the bow and in turn she also became frustrated.

As we had missed out on Morocco in 1991 we made reservations for Club Med in Marrakesh for February 1992. This time we made it. While Mary seemed to enjoy many things on the trip I was totally unable to leave her to do anything by herself. At the same time she related to others and most did not recognize that she had any problem.

In 1992 we went to Seattle for the wedding of Mary's niece Barbara. Mary's brother Bill lent us a car and we had a short trip round the Olympia National Park. Everything went well on our three days in the National Park; however another serious problem arose on our return trip to Philadelphia. For some reason the flight was Seattle to San Francisco then changing planes for Los Angles and changing again for Philadelphia. In San Francisco Mary needed to go to the toilet. I was not watching and she apparently came out of the toilet and wandered off. I certainly had some anxious moments until I eventually found her.

At another time Mary entered a woman's toilet and apparently was unable to find her way out. On that occasion a woman we happened to know passed by and I asked her to go into the toilet and find Mary. After those episodes, I had to restrict where I took Mary. By the end of 1993 she could not go to any public toilet by herself.

Our final trip together was in September 1994. I had to attend a conference in Seattle. We went together and Mary was able to stay with her brother, Bill, while I spent several days at the hotel where the conference was being held. Things went reasonably well, but Bill complained that he was not able to carry on a conversation with Mary. At least at that time she was able to answer when she was spoken to. This also shows that even close relatives don't understand the difficulties with the Alzheimer's patient.

CHAPTER 12

LEGAL PLANNING

We realized we had to plan. Unfortunately much of what we learned was by chance. In the late 1980s Alzheimer's disease was not widely discussed and few people were sufficiently informed to make the essential plans. It is hoped that persons reading this book will come to know that there are things that <u>can</u> and <u>must</u> be done <u>sooner</u> rather than later in order to lessen problems which <u>will</u> arise later as the disease progresses.

The essential planning is complicated by the fact that the patient, in the early stages of Alzheimer' disease insists that there is nothing wrong with them and resists giving up any control of their life or financial assets. We have already seen how most persons suffering from Alzheimer's resist giving up their car and the problem is worse with money and other possessions.

Another problem in completing the essential planning is that some members of the family may disagree as to what should be done and are reluctant to agree to another member taking control of the affairs of the patient. Often brothers or sisters, sons or daughters fail to understand the severity of the disease and its inevitable course. One man in a support group remarked that his daughter said to him "Dad I don't know what you are doing for mother, she is not getting any better!"

Lack of agreement as to how serious is the patient's condition frequently prevents the implementation of essential legal measures. Fortunately all members of Mary's family agreed on the severity of her condition but because of lack of knowledge, many legal measures which could have been implemented as soon as Alzheimer's disease was diagnosed were left too late with serious adverse consequences.

Families who wish to ease the burden of caring for a person with Alzheimer's disease should start planning years ahead but of course few people ever expect this tragedy to affect them. In addition to the normal need for a will, we found there are the several major actions which will greatly ease later problems:

- Have a lawyer draw up a Durable General Power of Attorney.
- Have a lawyer prepare a "Living will" or whatever similar provision is available in the particular state. This is a document in which the patient clearly indicates in front of competent witnesses that they do not wish to be kept alive on life support systems nor should there be heroic measure to revive them in the event that they collapse. Obviously this document must be signed before dementia has progressed.
- Benefits are available through Social Security, Medicare, and Medicaid. The local chapter of the Alzheimer's Association will be able to advise as to lawyers who specialize in this area, and who will advise as to eligibility for benefits and long-term medical care.

If possible, take out insurance to provide for long-term health care. The feasibility of taking out this insurance will depend on the age of the person when the policy opened. It will of course be impossible to get this insurance after a person has been diagnosed as having Alzheimer's disease. Therefore it is suggested that the family look into obtaining a suitable insurance policy if they suspect Alzheimer's disease.

It was not until the middle of 1990 that our lawyer heard of Mary's condition. He immediately advised that a power of attorney and a living will be prepared. Without these two documents, signed by Mary when she was still competent, my problems would have been much greater. They were both signed by Mary and duly notarized in August 1990.

At the same time the lawyer recommended that our home should be transferred from joint ownership to my name. Again this proved to be a very important action. When I had to sell the home I was able to execute all documents without question at a time when it would have been impossible for Mary to sign anything.

The above are some of the important planning actions that we only learned about through default, at a time when the full implications of Alzheimer's disease were only just becoming known by experts, let alone the public at large. It cannot be too strongly emphasized that, at the first signs of dementia, the family should seek expert legal advice. Unfortunately many families go through a period of denial - "father is getting old and a little forgetful". Such an attitude leads to serious difficulties as the dementia progresses.

Chapter 13

TESTING MARY

As part of a research project, the University of Pennsylvania had performed the initial evaluation of Mary at no cost to the Minter family. Thus when we were approached in January 1989 by another researcher, Dr. Gary Gottlieb, who asked that Mary participate in a research project to evaluate a new drug for the treatment of Alzheimer's disease, we readily agreed.

Dr. Gottlieb was director of the Section of Geriatric Psychology at the Hospital of the University of Pennsylvania and was serving as Principal Investigator on a Phase Three Clinical Trial for a drug designated as HP 029 (an experimental medication developed by Hoechst-Roussel Pharmaceuticals). Day to day procedures were performed by Dr. Gottlieb's Research Assistant, a Registered Nurse.

Mary attended the special center on the outskirts of the university campus on a monthly basis. This center, designed for the care of geriatric patients was located away from the hospital. Thus Mary was not intimidated by thinking she was returning to the hospital where they had discovered "the awful truth about her".

At the first meeting both of us were asked to sign a document acknowledging "informed consent". At that stage Mary may or may not have understood what she was being asked to sign. For people with Alzheimer's disease the matter of a patient granting "Informed Consent", for anything, is somewhat questionable. When do they still understand an abstract concept and when are they just "going along" with what they are being asked to do? Mary went through a series of tests which included both interviews and medical screening to establish a base-line.

The informed consent form stated that the subject may be receiving the drug or receiving a placebo. It also pointed out that this drug had already gone through a series of tests in both young and in elderly healthy men. It went on to state that "When patients with Alzheimer's Disease were given the doses of HP 029 some of them had cramps, nausea, vomiting, teary eyes, a runny nose, depression and hostility". In fact at least the last three symptoms can be seen frequently in almost all Alzheimer's patients, even if they are not receiving any medication. However, the significant side effect stated on the form was "Some patients taking HP 029 had damage to the liver while taking the drug." For that reason Mary had to have a blood test on each visit to the research center. Drawing the blood was the only aspect of the study she objected to. Fortunately by the time we returned for each monthly visit she had forgotten about having blood drawn until it was time to have it done. Therefore during this trial there was little problem in getting her to the research center and gaining her cooperation.

At each visit, of about one and a half hours, the following three activities were completed:

- Mary received a medical evaluation
- Mary was questioned about things such as what day it was, what season of the year, or where she was. She was also asked to count backwards from 100 by numbers such as seven. That is 93, 86, 79, etc. - not easy even for people in good mental condition. At first she was able to answer most of the questions but as the trial progressed she was less able to respond. She was also asked to draw geometric figures.
- I, as designated care giver, was asked to complete a questionnaire concerning Mary's condition and activities over the previous month.

At the conclusion of each session, the research assistant gave me a vial of pills which were always more than the number needed for 30 days in case it was not possible for Mary to have an appointment exactly 30 days later. On returning for the next appointment the number of pills remaining were carefully counted and recorded.

Actually, while neither the researchers nor I knew whether Mary was receiving the drug or the placebo, the dosage level was supposed to be changing each month. In fact I believe that at least for some months she did actually receive the drug while on other months she probably received the placebo. In this way the researchers were able to assess any differences in her condition and response to tests from month to month and relate any differences to whether she was receiving the drug or the placebo during the previous month.

I did consider that some months she showed improvement and on other months she seemed to slip back. However, such changes in the short term are consistent with most persons with Alzheimer's disease even if they are not receiving medication. At the conclusion of the trial no further information was made available to us and as far as is known HP 029 never did receive FDA approval.

By November 1989 the Section of Geriatric Psychiatry had another research project and again Mary was asked to participate. This project was a trial for a new product developed by E.R. Squibb & Sons Pharmaceuticals (now Bristol-Myers, Squibb). The product was SQ 29,852 and I was told that it was a modification of Squibb's ACE Inhibitor (an antihypertensive agent) Capoten. The objective of the study was indicated as "to determine the effectiveness and safety of different doses of SQ 29,852 in the treatment of patients with Alzheimer's disease." Mary was told that the study would last seven months and involve eight visits to the research center. During the study she was told that she would receive either a placebo or one of four different doses of the drug.

This trial was rather unique in that the participants were asked to respond to an interactive video program by touching the screen to indicate their response. Although I asked to view this video testing program, because of my professional interest in training, I was told that Squibb would not allow it. It would certainly seem that the concept of using an interactive video program for testing people who definitely have impaired ability to read and write is an excellent concept. The clinical trial proceeded as scheduled with Mary sometimes having a good month and at other times she seemed to be deteriorating. Again it was disappointing that we received no indication of whether she received the drug or a placebo and we were never given any indication of her results.

During the course of this second experiment, Mary was asked to participate in another special experiment conducted by a medical researcher, Dr. Deborah Beretta. She was studying the flow of blood in the brains of patients suffering from Alzheimer's disease. For this experiment, Mary was required to spend most of one day in the nuclear medicine center of the main University of Pennsylvania hospital. It did not seem to cause her any worry. However, later when Mary was being evaluated by Dr. Clark in 1996, I mentioned this special one-day experiment but no one at the university seemed to have heard of it. By that time Dr. Beretta had moved on to another hospital.

By February 1994 Mary was asked to participate in another clinical trial at the Section of Geriatric Psychiatry. This trial involved another drug from Hoechst Roussel Pharmaceuticals.

This time the drug had a generic name *besipirdine hydrochloride* as well as the experimental number HP 749. This trial was to run for 532 days and participants were seen every 2 to 4 weeks for a total of 27 visits. The protocol for this trial differed somewhat from that of the other two. During the first 6 months of the trial, participants received either of one of two different doses of the drug or a placebo. If the participant tolerated the first 6 months without adverse effects, then that person would definitely receive HP 749 during the next 48 weeks.

In addition to the blood tests and questionnaires answered by both the patients and the care giver, electrocardiograms were taken at 16 of the visits. Mary started out quite well but her condition deteriorated during the course of the trial. Also the principal investigator, Dr. Gary Gottlieb, left the University of Pennsylvania. His place was taken by Dr. Anand Kumar. Sometime after Mary entered phase two of this trial, when she was definitely receiving HP 749, she began to protest about going to the university. These protests became worse and eventually on one visit she was vicious and positively refused to get out of the car. Dr. Kumar had to go out to the car and beg her to go into the clinic so she could at least get a final blood test and EKG. Those final tests were essential to complete FDA requirements. Obviously Mary had to be dropped from that trial.

It was time consuming and moderately expensive to take Mary to the various sessions at the University of Pennsylvania, a trip of 25 miles each way. However, we considered it a public responsibility to assist the research that is needed to learn more about Alzheimer's disease. There was a very slight chance that one of the products may have helped Mary but a more important consideration was that a useful product may help others, even Mary's children, at a later date.

The first product approved by the FDA for the treatment of Alzheimer's disease was *tacrine hydrochloride* with the brand name COGNEX®. This is a reversible cholinesterase inhibitor which has been shown to slow the mental decline of the Alzheimer's disease patient. However warnings are given that, among other things, the product may lead to cardiovascular conditions, gastrointestinal dysfunction, and liver injury. Because of the possibility of liver damage, patients receiving COGNEX must have blood tests to monitor liver function. Since Mary was already seriously demented we decided not to subject her to the risk of adverse reactions.

After Mary was dropped from the HP 749 trial in the summer of 1994 she had no further medical attention until June 1996. Friends had been warning me that our daughters may have inherited a possibility of developing Alzheimer's. As will be explained in the next chapter, I had become involved in the work of the Alzheimer's Association of Southeastern Pennsylvania. I called Helen-Ann Comstock, the Association's Executive Director, and discussed this matter. Helen-Ann told me that Dr. Christopher Clark at the Memory Disorders Clinic at the Hospital of the University of Pennsylvania was conducting extensive research on the disease and particularly the relationship of early onset Alzheimer's disease (AD) to genes which affect apoprotein E (ApoE). An appointment was scheduled with Dr. Clark. It was quickly determined that, by that time, Mary was too far advanced to be able to participate in the particular trial. She would not have been able to respond to specific questions.

When Dr. Clark saw Mary he immediately determined that she was suffering from "Diffuse Lewy Body Disease." This is a variation of AD and is closely linked to Parkinson's disease. Lewy Bodies are eosinophilic inclusions which are usually found in the brainstem but sometimes in the cerebral cortex. I researched Diffuse Lewy Body Disease and found that a "Lewy Net" page had been established on the internet following a meeting of a consortium of clinicians and neuropathologists at Newcastle upon Tyne, UK, in October 1995.

Dr. Clark was able to detect the symptoms of Parkinson's disease in Mary from the way she walked and from the rigidity of her arms. Mary was not eligible to participate in the specific trial at The Memory Disorders Clinic, but because of the fact that she had received a very extensive medical evaluation at the University of Pennsylvania some eight years previously, Dr. Clark decided to undertake a follow-up review and copies of the original PET scans performed on Mary were located, some of the earliest PET (Positron Emission Tomography) scans used for the diagnosis of AD.

At future visits to the hospital, Mary had blood and spinal fluid drawn and permission was given for the hospital to store those samples for later comparison at the autopsy after her death. The spinal fluid was sent to Japan for evaluation. She also visited the Department of Nuclear Medicine where further PET scans were performed. The following is a copy of the report from Dr. Clark:

Mary's illness remains compatible with the general diagnosis of Alzheimer's disease. In addition, she has a moderate degree of Parkinsonism and may well have the Lewy body variant of Alzheimer's disease. This is a form of Alzheimer's disease which combines the gen-

eral pathological changes seen with that disorder with the pathological changes seen with Parkinson's disease. It is not simply the confluence of both of those clinical diseases in that these patients frequently do not have the typical Parkinson changes in their basal ganglion and rarely respond in a meaningful manner to standard Parkinson therapy.

I have reviewed the results of her recent PET scan and the comparison with her 1988 study. The initial study showed some subtle changes which were compatible with a clinical diagnosis of Alzheimer's disease. There were no changes in the basal ganglion. She has decreased metabolism in both parietal lobes, both temporal lobes, the occipital lobes, and, to a lesser extent, both frontal lobes. There were no significant changes in the basal ganglion or the subcortical nuclei.

Her ApoE genotype is 3/4. The presence of an ApoE4 is considered a risk factor for Alzheimer's disease, but is certainly not diagnostic of that condition. Since she has two first degree blood relatives who may also have had Alzheimer's disease, the condition could be said to be running in her family. She does not have a genetic form of Alzheimer's disease in that it is unlikely that a specific gene mutation is responsible for her illness. However, because of the nature of the family history, it is possible that each first degree relative in her family has up to a four-fold increased risk of Alzheimer's disease compared to persons who are members of a family for whom no blood relative is known to have been affected. This should have no practical impact as far as the members of your family are concerned, as even the presence of a four-fold increase should not be considered significant enough to change their long-term plans or modify the way they look at the future.

I do not yet have the results of Mary's spinal fluid tau or beta amyloid 1-42 levels. Both of these are research studies and have been sent to my colleague in Japan who performs the assay. Her routine spinal fluid values were normal. She had a protein of 33 and glucose of 59, with one white blood cell.

As a result of this further evaluation by the Memory Disorders Clinic, we agreed that, after Mary's death, the University of Pennsylvania should perform an autopsy so that the actual condition of her brain could be compared with the various test results. By examining the condition of her brain cells, researchers could correlate the findings to the clinical signs which had been revealed in the earlier examinations.

Chapter 14

CAREGIVING

Alzheimer's disease (AD) is one of the most taxing diseases from the point of view of the caregiver. It continues to tax the caregiver over a long period of time, usually at least for 5 years. Most significantly the disease takes away all that is essentially human in the patient. The care- giver never receives thanks from the patient and frequently is treated with hostility and abuse.

When my daughters and I received the news that Mary was suffering from AD we decided to tell Mary. It was one of the few times I recall when Mary broke down and cried. It is probable that she did not realize the full impact of her condition nor what it would mean in the years to come. Never-the-less she realized that it was something serious.

After receiving the diagnosis things in the household returned pretty much to normal. As I have explained, we were building a house and Mary threw herself into all the tasks involved. For the first few years following the diagnosis we continued with our social contacts and we continued to travel together.

A number of books have been written concerning the progress of Alzheimer's disease and its effects on the family. One of the best known is *The 36 Hour Day, Understanding Alzheimer's disease.* Another book written with more love and understanding is *Elegy for Iris* written by John Bailey. John is a literary critic who records the decline of his wife Iris Murdoch, a noted novelist.

While there are certain common aspects to the disease progression, each individual will have a different timing. The following table shows a scale of different stages in the progression of the disease and the approximate date when we believe Mary reached each stage.

Stage	Functional Ability	Reached Stage
1	No loss of functional ability either subjectively or objectively	1981
2	Complains of forgetting location of objects and may have subjective work difficulties	1985
3	Decreased functioning in demanding work and difficulty in traveling to new locations	1989
4	Decreased ability to perform complex tasks(reading books or magazines)	1991
5	Requires assistance in selecting clothes; unable to write more than her signature, and unable to drive	1992
6a	Difficulty dressing	May 1993
b	Fear of bathing, must have assistance	Aug. 1994
c	Difficulty with mechanics of toileting	Dec. 1994
d	Occasional fecal incontinence	Jan. 1996
e	Unable to sign her name	Mar. 1996
7a	Vocabulary limited to a few words	Apr. 1996
b	Intelligible vocabulary lost	Dec. 1996
c	Totally incontinent	Jan. 1997
d	Basically unable to feed herself	Mar. 1997
e	Unable to walk	Mar. 1997
f	Unable to sit	Did not reach
g	Unable to eat - whole food	Aug. 1998
h	Unable to drink normal liquids	Feb. 1999
i	Ultimate stupor or coma	Did not reach
j	Unable to swallow food or liquid	July 4, 1999
k	Death	July 7, 1999

There are the difficulties the caregiver experiences due to the actual condition of the patient and there are also the changes which must occur in the spouse's activities. For example, I had developed a successful business preparing training materials for Fortune 500 companies. As Mary's condition progressed, not only was I not able to devote my full time to servicing existing clients but I was not able to keep abreast of emerging technology such as computer assisted instruction. Consequently the company started to run down and eventually I had to sell out in the early months of 1994.

After closing a 10,000 square foot office I moved a limited office into the basement of our home. My secretary, who had worked with the company for 12 years, came to the home each day. Under this arrangement I continued to perform some consulting assignments and took on Directorship of The Australian Chamber of Commerce in Philadelphia. Attending to that work and having my secretary to talk with kept me from depression over the next four years as Mary became less and less responsive.

Like most husbands faced with caring for a wife with Alzheimer's disease, I was determined to look after Mary for as long as possible. The reasons for this were:

1 - It was the right thing to do;
2 - Nursing home care is so terribly expensive (at that time $50,000 to $75,000 per year.)

We hesitated to put Mary in a secure facility where she would be away from her home, and family and friends. However, it is advisable that research into options should be done sooner rather than when the need becomes painfully obvious. Price is a major consideration, as is comfort of patient, location of facility, and ability of facility to care for an Alzheimer patient.

At the end of 1992 I investigated other options for caring for Mary. There is no doubt that this investigation should have been done much earlier. I joined the Alzheimer's Association and reviewed their publications. These included lists of day care centers, in-home companion services, and full nursing homes which accepted patients with AD. Here is what I found:

Day Care:

> Several facilities which provided day care were located in counties surrounding our home. Some only accepted persons from the county, while others accepted persons from a wider area. It seemed that the closest centers were at least 10 miles from our home. I investigated them with Mary but she refused to attend them. Her main complaint was that the other people at the centers were sick or "crazy". At that time she certainly did not consider that there was anything the matter with her.
>
> Apart from Mary's rejection, the centers would not have been very practical. They accepted patients from 9 to 5 or 8 to 4 Monday through Friday. Two of them provided service on only 2 days per week. The fees at that time were $30 to$40 per day. For Mary to have attended one of these day care centers would have entailed my driving an additional 20 miles per day as well as cutting short my time at the office. At that time I still worked from the outside office.

In Home Care:

> Several organizations which provided visiting home nurses also had qualified persons who would "live in" during the week. The charges for this service were approximately $150 per day which was almost as much as full nursing home care. At the same time the family had to provide a room and food for the live-in attendant. This option may have been acceptable for a very wealthy family who already had a large home and a live-in servant but did not help greatly if the spouse had to look after the attendant. In fact it was only practical for short periods, if the spouse had to travel away for several days.

Nursing Homes:

> I visited several nursing homes near our home, some accepted AD patients, many did not. The prices were $150 to $160 per day and the facilities were excellent. But I did not consider Mary was ready for nursing home care at that time and with the expenses of owning a home I was not able to commit the funds for this sort of care.

Other Options:

I then asked our church if there were any retired women who might take Mary out for one or two days per week. Someone knew a woman, who attended another church, who would do that for $20 per hour plus lunch for both Mary and herself. By mid 1994 I decided that Mary should go with this woman for four hours on 2 days per week. That program continued through the end of 1994 and then I heard about a program which the Greater Philadelphia Chapter of the Alzheimer's Association was running in conjunction with the Manor Care nursing home (now HCR Manor Care) in the area. This program was known as the "Club". It took AD patients for 4 hours on two days per week. The facilities were excellent and a trained occupational therapist helped the patients with a wide range of activities.

HCR Manor Care, Inc., is a nation-wide corporation headquartered in Toledo, Ohio. They operate several hundred nursing homes across the United States which are organized into regional centers, such as the one at King of Prussia, Pennsylvania.

Before Mary was accepted for the Club, Judy Moss, the director for the Alzheimer's program in the Manor Care regional center needed to meet with her in our home. I was most impressed with Judy's professionalism. She had certainly studied the disease and at the time of our meeting had just returned from attending an International Conference on Alzheimer's disease which had been held in Scotland.

She determined that Mary was a suitable candidate for the Club, which was held from 10 am through 2 p.m. on Tuesdays and Thursdays. Members met in the conference room of the King of Prussia Manor Care home, had lunch together, and the occupational therapist organized structured activities. The fee was $20 per day.

Mary seemed to enjoy this program, so the arrangement with the woman who took Mary out twice per week was terminated. However, about that time two women from our church volunteered to take Mary out for lunch for a further two days per week. Thus I was free from cares about Mary during the middle of the day on four days per week.

During the rest of the time, I did practically everything for Mary. Fortunately Mary did not have trouble sleeping. In fact at that time, Mary did not exhibit the following problems which are often mentioned as being common with the Alzheimer's patient:

- She did not wander. We lived on 6 acres and the road was a quarter of a mile from the home, so she would have needed to go a long way before reaching the road. She certainly could have gone away from the home but she never once did so.
- She did not seem to have a problem with losing things. If things were mislaid that certainly did not lead Mary to worry about them.
- She never accused anyone of stealing her possessions.
- She never hallucinated.
- She always behaved appropriately for the occasion.
- She did not break things.
- She usually did not turn on the stove and leave it on, although occasionally she did leave the water running. At one time she turned on the water in the laundry tub when the plug was in the drain and it overflowed. The laundry was on the main floor and of course the water poured through to the basement making a terrible mess. This did not occur again as I continued to turn the water off at the valve.

CHAPTER 15

A ROUTINE DEVELOPS

As I have said Mary usually slept well. At 6 am I got up and shaved. Then I turned on the shower and got Mary out of her night dress. By mid 1994 she had come to dislike water or bathing. Left to her own she claimed, "I just had a bath". I found that there were only two ways to beat this. We had a Jacuzzi bath large enough for both of us. So at least once a week I would fill the Jacuzzi and put in bubble bath. Then we would both climb in and let it bubble away for 15 minutes. I got out first, dried off, and got into my pajamas before getting Mary out and dried. On weekday mornings the only way to get Mary bathed was for me to take my shower with her. Again this required a careful routine. I put out Mary's towel, put a shower cap on her and we both got in the shower together. I soaped Mary and washed her off then she dried herself while I showered. Since there was an infra-red strip heater in the bathroom I was able to leave Mary while I dressed. Then I dressed her. At first this was just a matter of getting Mary's clothes ready for her but later I needed to put everything on her.

Mary often tried to do things herself but it soon became evident that letting her perform the task was a lot more trouble than doing it by myself. One such task was making the bed. If I did not do this, the bed always ended up a mess. At first it was possible for me to supervise bed making with Mary on the other side pulling up sheets and straightening them, but later that became unsatisfactory.

When Mary was no longer able to help with the task, I left the bed making until after breakfast. I prepared cereal and fruit and made coffee and toast. While Mary was eating I went back to the bedroom and made the bed.

Even though Mary was not able to dress herself, she had strong opinions as to what she should wear. Frequently I would have her dressed and through breakfast, only to find that after I had gone down to my office in the basement,

Mary had changed into something completely different. This was most difficult as she only half dressed herself in the new outfit and had to be re-dressed.

This routine continued satisfactorily for a few months with changes from day to day. Some days Mary would be very cooperative and everything went well. Other days she became very belligerent and wanted to fight. Unfortunately as a result of this I sometimes reacted and became very annoyed. After all I was doing for her it was just too much to have her fight me. This seems to be a universal experience of caregivers working with Alzheimer's patients.

Early in 1996 I had gone down to my office right after breakfast and left Mary still eating in the kitchen. Later on coming up stairs I was aware of an odor. I found that Mary had apparently had a bowel movement in her pants and then taken them off. The fecal matter had dropped on the bathroom floor, then Mary had stepped in it and walked round the house. Considering the fact that our carpets were off-white, you can imagine the cleaning problem. On two other occasions it happened when the realtor was bringing prospective buyers to look at the house.

In 1995 I was the recipient of the Terry McGill award for the person who had done the most to further Australian American relations during the previous year. The ceremony took place in the Grand Ballroom of the Plaza Hotel in New York City on Australia Day, January 26th. Mary and Margaret were present. That was the last occasion on which Mary and I were able to attend a formal dinner together.

The following year, 1996, I was asked to be present when the award was passed to the new recipient. By that stage it was not possible for Mary to go to such an event. Manor Care Nursing Home provided "Respite Care" for caregivers, so I arranged for Mary to go into the nursing home for two days. After lunch I packed a bag with Mary's clothes for overnight and set off in the car for the nursing home. No mention of the plans was made to Mary.

Even though she was going to the facility where she attended the "Club" on two days per week, she became uneasy as we approached the facility. When we stopped at the nursing home, she refused to get out of the car. Then when I finally did get her out of the car she took off out of the parking area at a great pace. Fortunately I managed to turn her round and head her in the door. There we were met by the director of admissions who immediately took us down to the Arcadia Unit, which is the part of the nursing home reserved for Alzheimer's patients. This area is secured by locks operated by key pads so once in that area she was safe. I left immediately while Mary screamed.

When I returned for Mary the next day she was participating in one of the group activities and did not seem to want to leave. This was my first clear indication that the nursing home environment was not going to be so bad for her. In May of 1996 the management of Manor Care asked me if I would go to Harrisburg to speak to a committee of the Pennsylvania Department of Health in support of the construction of a new Nursing Home in Chester County, the county in which we lived. In return for this support, Manor Care agreed to take Mary into the Arcadia Unit for a further two days. This time there was some, but not as much, trouble getting Mary into the facility, and again she was not anxious to leave when I returned to collect her.

During this time we continued to go to social events whenever possible. On a Saturday in early June I was asked to a garden party. It was a beautiful day, sunny with a light breeze and moderate temperature. In the early part of the afternoon I had to sit in on a meeting at the facility where the party was being held, so I left Mary sitting with several other women on lawn chairs. At that time she hardly was able to speak so she did not get a drink or any food. When I returned a crowd had gathered and I got a drink and some food for Mary. Then she suddenly threw back her head, went pale and after gasping a little seemed to stop breathing. There was a doctor in the crowd so he came over but she then seemed to start breathing again. About eighteen months later she had a similar turn while she was in the Arden Courts assisted living facility.

After this attack at the garden party the doctor said he thought she had been sitting in the sun for too long and was dehydrated. We gave her a long drink and I drove her home. She still did not seem well so I put her to bed. When I walked back into the bedroom she had vomited!

Just one day in the life of a caregiver...

CHAPTER 16

NURSING HOME DECISIONS

Mary was becoming more difficult to handle. There was almost nothing that could be done to keep her entertained. During the early months of 1996 she constantly walked round with a copy of Sherlock Holmes. Sometime she would sit for hours staring at it. Sometimes the book was upside down but it seemed to her that it was appropriate for her to appear to others that she was doing something meaningful. In the end the Sherlock Holmes book was totally worn out.

During the early part of 1996 Manor Health Care Inc. developed a new concept for persons with early stage Alzheimer's disease - units named *Arden Courts*. One of these units was opened at the Manor Care facility in King of Prussia, PA.

That particular unit had a central administration and activity area with a square hallway surrounding it. At the four corners of the square there were living units. Each living unit consisted of hallways leading to a kitchen / dining area. On either side of the hallways were individual rooms, each with a private bathroom. Each of the four corner units was self contained and accommodated about 15 residents. Units were decorated in different colors and named, "Peach Tree Court"; "Blue Spruce Circle" etc. This made it easy for the residents to recognize their own area. The whole Arden Court complex was like a large ranch house. Inside, the appearance was extremely bright and refreshing.

By July 1996 our home was under contract for sale. Therefore the girls and I decided to immediately place Mary in Arden Courts so we could pack up the household items and have a monster garage sale. Had Mary been in the home at that time she would not only have been disruptive to the efforts but would have suffered a great deal of trauma in seeing her home being taken apart.

The family elected to only provide a limited number of pictures and some knick-knacks for her room. The rooms of some residents were fitted out with fine furniture and TV sets. As Mary had long since ceased to watch TV that was not needed. I visited her each evening for the first few weeks. Actually she settled in remarkably well. Never once did she want to go home. However on every visit she would earnestly ask "what are you doing?" The living quarters did not seem to upset Mary, but for the first week or so I went home in tears at having to leave her at Arden Courts.

The front door into the complex was secured and had to be opened with a key pad. Outside the building was an extensive garden area with lawns, flower beds and walk ways. This open area was enclosed with a high chain link fence and one could only enter or leave the garden by way of the actual home itself. Patients were able to walk around the garden on nice days and could go in or out of their residential area as they wished.

The fact that residents were virtually kept under lock and key was important to the welfare of the individuals but a problem with legal implications. On one occasion an executive of Manor Health Care Corp., when speaking with a meeting of care givers of the patients in Arden Courts, indicated that the company had spent nearly $100,000 in Pennsylvania getting permission to keep Alzheimer's patients in a secure facility. He also said that in another state they had been told that they were not able to construct "jails". Further problems arise when people associated with the "Americans with Disabilities" movement become involved. It seems to me that some people have absolutely no concept of how Alzheimer's patients behave.

It is very clear that people who have been diagnosed with Alzheimer's disease will at some time wander from their environment and become lost or even severely injured. It is also clear that the same people will have days on which they will claim that they are being kept against their will.

During the days when I sat with Mary and helped her eat, I was able to make some interesting observations about the group of patients in the unit.

On one occasion I met a sprightly elderly woman whom I had not seen previously. She walked up and said that she needed to visit a bank and would I please give her directions to the nearest one. Thinking she was a visitor, I took care to describe how she should drive out of the parking lot turn right and then left at the next intersection, and so on. Several days later I saw the same woman again and she was just jabbering unintelligibly.

Another woman I saw regularly was a member of a well known wealthy family from Ohio, and was a graduate of Smith College. For some reason, that woman thought I was a lawyer. Every time she saw me she rushed up and asked me to take out proceedings against Manor Care for keeping her against her will.

Another woman, from Pittsfield, Mass. was 89 but looked to be hardly more than 70. She was also a graduate of Smith. To her everything was always so beautiful - the day, the clouds, the flowers, etc. She could carry on a reasonable conversation and was most pleasant although always saying that she had "been sick and her doctor had advised he to stay at Arden Courts for a while but she was going home shortly".

In the same unit there was a woman for whom everything was wrong. At mealtime she would always say they had given her much more food than she could eat and she was not going to pay for all that wasted food. On a number of occasions she would come to me and ask me to get her a suppository! In other respects that woman was often able to speak quite intelligently.

Two other women in the same unit were quite different in their level of ability. One was only able to make noises such as "blub, blub, etc." and the other seemed to be absolutely unable to speak. That woman was quiet; she looked at people with intensity and a glint in her eyes. Her mouth would tremble and on many occasions she would appear to cry quietly. She was virtually unable to feed herself any time I observed her. It shows the range of different ways in which the disease can affect different people.

On the other hand, there was one woman who used to take her spoon or fork and tap out a tune on her plate. The woman was quite musical, but the other patients used to get very upset and would yell for her to stop.

When first admitted to Arden Courts, Mary was able to speak reasonably coherently and was able to feed herself. She was only occasionally experiencing incontinence and was bathing without much effort. It was difficult to get her to have her hair washed but I sometimes took her to Elizabeth's home where they would get it washed with only limited trouble. I used to go to Arden Courts after dinner and, while the weather was warm, we would both walk round the grounds. Then I would clean Mary's teeth and dental floss them. Usually that was accomplished without great difficulty. Finally I would put her into bed and read to her.

The food at Arden Courts was quite good. At first the juice was Kool-Aid. However at a meeting of care givers there were strong complaints about the quality of the drinks so that following that meeting the management provided real juices. Even though the food was good and Mary appeared to be feeding herself, her weight dropped. On entering Arden Courts she weighed 165 lbs. By the end of 1996 she was down to only 132 lbs.

Obviously the loss concerned the nurses at Arden Courts and she was put on a high calorie diet but she never regained weight. To guard against Mary not eating, I attempted to be present for at least one meal each day. She could still use a spoon and fork but she usually ate by picking up the food in her hands, and pushing it into her mouth. However by about November of 1996 she had lost the ability to use a spoon or fork.

LIFE IN REVERSE...

CHAPTER 17

MOOD SWINGS AND DECLINE

During the latter part of 1996 Mary's condition went through marked changes. Sometimes she was most difficult and at other times she was bright and cooperative. Friends made a point of saying "she seems very good, she understands me and there seems to be little wrong with her." Obviously they did not see her at her bad times! This is one of the serious problems with Alzheimer's; Mary experienced some extreme mood swings.

In September 1996, I had a friend from Australia staying with me and I took him along one day when I visited Mary. We spotted some sort of scratching in one of the flower beds when the three of us were walking round the garden, probably made by a rabbit. We looked at this and Mary said, "what did that?" The Australian said "probably a kangaroo" Mary laughed heartily at that statement – a moment of apparent clarity?

While Mary was able to speak only in single sentences when she entered Arden Courts, she lost practically all ability to talk by the end of the year. From time to time when she would get agitated she would repeat "bugger, bugger, bugger". Strangely, while I was sitting with Mary during meals I noticed that other patients would repeat the same thing or mumbling something very close to "bugger, bugger."

One day in mid-November when I visited Mary, she did not seem to recognize me and ordered me out of her room. During this latter part of 1996, Elizabeth and I tried to take Mary to church services as often as possible. These occasions were usually OK but it was getting increasingly difficult to get Mary up to the communion rail in the church; and once there she usually did not understand that she needed to kneel. The priests and everyone else were very understanding but it was obviously getting more and more difficult and also a distraction to others.

In early December, I was assigned to carry the chalice for the communion service so I asked a friend to help Mary up to the rail. With difficulty the friend managed to get her up and, even though the priest placed the wafer into her mouth, she refused to eat it.

The following week was the 90th birthday of a church member who was one of our special friends, and I arranged to take Mary to the celebration. On arrival at Arden Courts I found that Mary was refusing to eat breakfast. Eventually I got her to drink orange juice, and eat some cereal but she refused to take her anti-hypertensive pills, just spat them out. I pushed ahead with my plan to get Mary to the birthday reception and by the time we got there she was sweetness and light and spoke very lovingly to the man whose birthday we were celebrating.

Here is another case where Mary appeared to be totally disoriented and then related to something with insight. By mid-December, Mary was leaning mark-edly to one side. The lean was so great that it was amazing she could continue to stand. While in the car taking Mary to church she continued to lean while secured by her seat belt. In fact she was so far over me that I had difficulty driv-ing. Once we arrived in the church she seemed totally confused and had diffi-culty walking. The priest, originally from Canada, preached on Christmases past.

He recalled the Christmas of 1936 when he was a young boy in the church choir. He said, "They sang 'Hark the Herald Angels Sing, Mrs. Simpson stole our King'". At that Mary was one of the first to burst out laughing. Mary's mother often spoke with great hatred of Mrs. Simpson who had pursued King Edward. Even with Alzheimer's Mary fully understood the historical incident.

That Mary was able to understand the humor in the priest's statement not only took memory, but also the intellectual ability to relate to the context. Did Mary understand this or was she just laughing because it seemed funny? If others had laughed first and Mary had followed, then we could assume that she was just laughing because others laughed, but it seemed apparent that Mary was the first to understand the humor. That was the last time Mary was able to attend church.

On December 17, 1996 one of the nurses from Arden Court phoned to say that Mary had collapsed. Apparently she was walking in the hallway with one of the nurses when she sank to the floor. She had stopped breathing and the nurse was unable to detect a heartbeat. This condition continued for about two minutes and the nurses were about to have Mary carried to her bed and phone me to make funeral arrangements. Then Mary opened her eyes and commenced breathing. The nurse then called 911 and had an ambulance take Mary to the emergency room at the local hospital.

After phoning our daughters, I went to the hospital. On arrival, I found Mary on a gurney with an IV drip in her hand, two lab workers were attempting to draw blood but were unable to locate a vein. X-rays and an EKG had been taken. I had to go through the procedure for admission and give all medical insurance information. The doctor in charge suggested that it would take some time to get results, so I returned to my office and phoned the hospital every hour. Eventually, about 5 p.m. the doctor said he could find nothing wrong with Mary and she definitely had not had a heart attack. By that time she was extremely difficult and did not want to cooperate in anything including getting into the car to return to Arden Courts. She kept saying "you get out of here".

It is this characteristic of the Alzheimer's patient that is so difficult for the care giver to handle. At the same time this difficult behavior is usually not apparent to persons who are not so close to the patient. That is, friends and relatives often don't see this aspect of the patient's behavior. They only see them in their quieter and friendlier moments, and so cannot understand why the care giver has any difficulty.

On this occasion, once in the car with the radio on, there was some mention of the University of Wisconsin and Mary immediately pricked up her ears to see what that was about - very strange how she recognized Wisconsin and changed her attitude immediately.

Arden Courts management asked me to meet with their consultant psychiatrist, Dr. Seara. He said that the Parkinson's disease was leading to stiffness and Mary's way of manifesting the problems was to adopt the leaning position. Attendants at the home were worried that she would fall but the doctor believed she was perfectly stable and would not fall unless she again became unconscious. He went on to say that if we treated the Parkinson's disease it would probably increase her agitation and then she would need sedation which in turn would only make her weaker and more likely to fall.

All in all he preferred not to treat the Parkinson's disease. He pointed out that she would probably continue to have the syncope attacks and he was pleased to know that I had a "do not resuscitate order" with Arden Courts. He also suggested that in future incidents there was little point in them phoning the rescue squad.

Dr. Seara then went on to point out that "assisted living", as provided at Arden Courts, was not then appropriate for Mary. He said that even if food is placed in front of her she was not able to eat it. One point he made was not to take Mary by the hand and try to draw her along that only caused her to resist. It was far better to place an arm round her and ease her in the direction she had to go.

Two days before Christmas one of the attendants at Arden Courts phoned to say that Mary had been incontinent and would not allow anyone to touch her. I left immediately for the nursing home with Margaret, who happened to be staying with me for Christmas. We found Mary wandering the hallway and smelled an odor right away. She perked up on seeing us and I led her to the bathroom. However, on realizing she was to have a bath she turned and ran. When I stopped her and turned her back to the bathroom she started screaming. I then got her undressed and into the bath.

After several minutes in the shower, Mary calmed down; I kissed her and dried her off. She then had a good lunch and Margaret and I left her in quite good spirits. Mary was not well enough to join the family at Elizabeth's home for Christmas Day 1996.

On the afternoon of the 29th of December, Arden Courts phoned to say that Mary was being difficult and would not allow anyone to touch her. When Margaret and I arrived Mary was wandering the hall as usual, in her night dress with only one shoe. I hugged her and took her back to her room where I was able to dress her. The attendants had kept her lunch in the refrigerator so I fed it to her. This was a very lengthy procedure as she did not appear very interested in food.

One thing I noticed was that on each occasion when Mary was agitated and refusing to do anything, she was very thirsty. One time she gulped down at least five glasses of juice. I passed on this information to the attendants and they took more care to see that Mary was drinking frequently. After that she seemed to improve.

These mood swings continued throughout the end of December, 1996 and early January 1997. On December 31st, 1996 the attendants phoned to say Mary was again not allowing anyone to dress her. I went to the home, got her dressed and fed her. The next day Elizabeth and I arrived at Arden Courts and were told that Mary was "great", very cooperative. They had got her into the shower and washed her hair.

Sometime during the night of January 9th, 1997 Mary must have fallen. In the morning the attendants found her sitting on the side of her bed with a gash above her right eye and a small cut on her nose. The nurse found blood on the floor by the bed-side table. It was assumed that Mary had hit her head on the edge of the table. On that occasion there was an icy rain so I was not able to go to see her.

When I arrived the next day Mary had the worst black eye I have ever seen. Now rather than walking with a lean to one side, she was walking with her head down on her chest while at the same time leaning forward. With her head down on her chest, it was only with extreme difficulty that I was able to feed her. It was practically impossible to get her mouth open and liquid would not run down her throat. This condition persisted for several days.

By the middle of January she was showing good improvement and was able to walk upright. However, the next day she was very restless and kept ordering me, "you get out of here!" The day following that the nurses said she had been "very good". What I am trying to stress is that these almost daily mood swings from violent antagonism to sweet cooperation are typical of the Alzheimer's patient and middle to late stage of the disease.

It was planned that Margaret and I would visit Australia during March 1997, so, because of Dr. Seara's comments that Mary was beyond the level of care which was available at Arden Courts, plans had to be made to cover emergencies while we were away.

First, considering the fact that Mary might die while we were away and that Elizabeth might also be away on a trip, funeral arrangements should be in place. In fact, these funeral arrangements should have been made much earlier. It is my recommendation that families should organize, sooner rather than later, and plan for what is to be done when the Alzheimer's patient eventually dies: choose a funeral director, who will help you with burial details and arrange for autopsy and organ donations.

Next consideration was that Mary was definitely deteriorating and had by then become totally incontinent and probably unable to feed herself while I was away. The "assisted living" level of care at Arden Courts did not allow for more than minimal assistance with feeding. Also things could become very difficult if the staff at Arden Courts were unable to bathe her, therefore it was decided to transfer her to the Arcadia Unit in the main Manor Care nursing home commencing on February 1, to allow a period for Mary to adjust prior to my departure. The Arcadia Unit is in the basement of the main facility and at that time was rather dark and dismal but they did have a more extensive and better trained staff that could feed the patients and bathe them.

For the rest of February I visited Mary at mealtimes and was able to observe the other patients. Only a few were able to carry on meaningful, although not very intelligent conversations, some needed walkers, and a few had wheel chairs, about 25% needed to be fed. A few, while still ambulatory, were almost totally unable to relate to anything. Mary seemed to fit in and certainly did not complain. She continued to walk up and down the corridor. While I was away in March everything seemed to go well and Elizabeth was able to visit her mother occasionally.

Upon returning to Philadelphia, I evaluated the situation and decided it was much more pleasant in Arden Courts and it was approximately $2,000 per month less expensive. Also the Arcadia Unit was scheduled for complete renovation, so I requested that Mary should return to Arden Courts in April 1997. This time I elected to have her in a semi-private room (2 persons). It was a slightly lower price than a single room and considering Mary's condition at that time, it was unlikely that another person in the room would affect her.

In fact during the period from April through the end of September when Mary was in the double room at Arden Courts a second woman was admitted to the room for only about 4 days. She died there on the fourth day. It is difficult to say whether that death was due to the fact that she was too far advanced when her care giver decided to admit her, that the shock of being institutionalized was too much for her, or whether she had some other condition in addition to Alzheimer's disease.

On the morning of April 12, 1997 (a Saturday), I received a call from the nurse on duty at Arden Courts informing me that Mary had fallen and was "in a mess". In compliance with my instructions they had not called 911 but I was told that I should get to Arden Courts as soon as possible. Mary indeed was in a mess. Apparently she had a syncope attack while walking in the corridor of her unit. In falling she hit her eye on the hand rail on the right side of the corridor. That eye was severely gashed. She appeared to have then rolled to the left and put her front teeth through her upper lip. The center two front teeth on the top jaw were loose and moving in the jaw.

I took her to the emergency room at the local hospital and admitted her. The doctor on duty did relevant checks and then put five stitches in her eye. Saturday was a light day at the hospital so they kept Mary and went through a lot of other checks. It was obvious that something needed to be done with her teeth but there was no dentist on duty. I spent most of the day at the hospital with her and then the doctor decided that she should remain in the hospital overnight.

I returned the next morning and drove her back to Arden Courts. At that time she was black and blue all over her entire face.

On Monday, I made an appointment with Mary's dentist and was able to take her to him that same afternoon. The dentist did not have a nurse or dental assistant, so I assisted by holding Mary down while he extracted the two front teeth. This was a gruesome experience. The poor woman did not know what was going on and continued to scream at the top of her lungs. The dentist decided to leave the third tooth that had been injured in the fall in the hope that it might last. Mary was to return for a check in a week.

During that week, the third injured tooth, which had a crown, broke off, leaving only the root at the gum line. Thus on the second visit the dentist had to dig out the root. This was also a very traumatic procedure. Everything considered, the dentist decided that it would probably be better for Mary not to have a denture. There was a possibility that she might swallow it.

The two visits to the hospital emergency room and the dental work that resulted from the fall highlighted problems with the Medicare coverage from Aetna-U.S. Health Care. Several weeks after both admissions a notice of refusal of coverage was received. It stated that coverage was denied because the primary care physician had not authorized hospital care.

In returning this notice, I pointed out that since Mary was in a nursing home and under constant care of the primary care physician assigned to that nursing home it would be impossible for Mary to go to a hospital emergency room without the knowledge of the primary care physician. That information was completely ignored when the insurers sent the same notice after the second visit to the emergency room. This sort of bureaucracy not only increases the paper work and cost for the insurance company but also increases the effort required by the already taxed caregiver. The final problem in the whole episode was that while Mary's coverage included limited dental care, they refused to cover the cost of the teeth removal, a medical necessity resulting from the fall, and would presumably have been covered in the total cost for the hospital emergency treatment had a dentist been available on the Saturday when Mary was admitted. Again a lot of time and paperwork were expended in trying to resolve this.

Back in Arden Courts, Mary continued through the summer of 1997 with the usual ups and downs. There were no further calls from management to say that Mary had fallen or that it was not possible to handle her. I continued to visit the facility for either lunch or dinner at least 3 or 4 times per week. Approximately every week Elizabeth and I went together and washed Mary's hair.

CHAPTER 18

BACK TO ARCADIA

In August the director of Arden Courts told me that Mary was beyond the level that was suitable for their facility and she would have to be transferred back to the Arcadia Unit in the main nursing home. Since renovations were still in progress it was decided to leave the transfer until October. Mary was finally re-admitted to the Arcadia Unit on October 1, 1997.

Things in the Arcadia Unit were pretty much the same as when Mary had left in March. There was new paint, new carpet and some re-arrangement of public areas. There were some new faces and some who were there in March had gone. Mary did not appear to realize she had moved from Arden Courts, at least she never tried to indicate that anything was different for her. Both the occupational therapists and the chaplain said on a number of occasions that "Mary seems to be participating more in the activities".

Mary still seemed to wander as much as she did in Arden Courts. Wander is possibly not the right word. When she was disturbed she would turn and take off at high speed. At other times she would just walk slowly up and down the one corridor in the unit. Every time I arrived to see her she would brighten up and sometimes put her arms round me and kiss me. However on almost every one of those visits she would get impatient and want to rush off. If I tried to clean her teeth she would fly into a rage, contort her face and strike out with her arms while yelling "you get out of here". I considered that it was important to try to keep her teeth in as good a condition as possible, especially as she had now lost three from the front of her mouth. At times while eating she would lapse into repeating "Bugger, Bugger, and Bugger" as she had been doing for the past 8 months or so.

Mary was in a double room at Arcadia and the companions changed from time to time either because they moved elsewhere or because they died.

Sometimes these companions were able to talk but at other times they did not. However, Mary was now essentially unable to talk. She often looked bright with a smile and frequently responded when spoken to. For that reason, visitors who had not seen her for some time, used to say, "She still understands" or "I don't think she is too bad". At other times she would be very difficult and scream when someone was trying to help her.

While a person in sound mind would feel confined in a situation such as this secure nursing home and might be even more concerned at having to share the room with another person, I am certain that Mary was unaware of her situation. In fact, after the first few days in Arden Court in 1996 she never ever asked to be taken home and did not seem concerned when we returned her to her room after she had been out to visit Elizabeth.

After October 1997 Mary was virtually unable to feed herself. A number of other residents in the Arcadia Unit were kept in a large reclining type of chair with wheels and had to be pushed from place to place. Others were in a frame type of chair, also with wheels, but in this case the patient's feet touched the floor so that they "walked" the chair about.

However through the rest of 1997 and most of 1998 Mary was mobile. In fact whenever we arrived at the nursing home she was still walking rapidly up and down the corridors. She continued to lose weight, possibly as a result of all this exercise. When she had entered Arden Courts she weighed 165 pounds. On entering the Arcadia she was about 120 pounds and by the time she was unable to walk at the end of 1998 she was down to about 90 pounds.

I was trying to ensure that Mary's remaining teeth would last as long as possible so, whenever I was with her for a meal, I used to take her to the bathroom and clean her teeth as well as I could. As the months went on teeth cleaning became more difficult. I had discontinued dental flossing when she left Arden Courts. By the middle of 1998 she seemed unable to spit out the rinse water after I had finished brushing. Sometime after January 1999 when she was essentially confined to the chair I had to discontinue teeth cleaning and was only able to wipe her mouth and teeth with a sponge on a stick.

After she transferred to the Arcadia Unit, I kept a running log of incidents in which Mary was involved. To give some feeling of the day-to-day events in the terminal months of a person with Alzheimer's disease I am sharing incidents as they happened.

CHAPTER 19

MY NURSING HOME LOG - 1997

October 31:

On arrival at the Arcadia Unit, I met Mary wandering in the hall. She beamed, put her arms around me and kissed me. We ate lunch together but when she was nearly finished she jumped up and wanted to leave. I went after her and tried to get her to clean her teeth. She flew into a rage, contorted her face, lashed out with her hands in a claw-like pose, and yelled "you get out of here".

November 4:

Mary was again walking in the hall and as I went up to her she kissed me. She was so cold that I went and got her a sweater and she cooperated in putting it on. I then noticed that there was another patient now in her room. We went into the dining room and I fed Mary her lunch. At the same time I brought out a card from her brother Bill and read it to her. She seemed to understand who Bill was. All-in-all she was quite cooperative over lunch and finished all I gave her.

Then we went and I cleaned her teeth which had not been cleaned since October 31. While we were in the bathroom, rinsing her mouth, one of the men patients walked in and started to urinate in the toilet. An action such as that is not unusual for a man suffering with Alzheimer's disease, but Mary did not seem to notice it. As I was leaving we kissed and Mary said "thank you". This was the first time in ages and probably the last time that she said "thank you".

November 7:

I received a phone call from Manor Care about 3 p.m. to say that Mary had fallen again. This time she had hit the back of her head, apparently on the hand rail by the nurse's quarters. Again they had no knowledge of how she had fallen. I arrived at about 4.45 p.m. and met with Jill Sobel the Director. Mary had a very small lump and was still walking rapidly along the corridor. I noticed that her mouth was caked with dried saliva and her teeth were covered with a scum. As I was not able to find her tooth brush and tooth paste, Jill called one of the men attendants and had him clean her teeth.

About 10 p.m. I received another call from Manor Care. The woman said "your mom has been in a fight with one of the men". Apparently the man punched her in the nose and she had a cut but the woman said she was O.K. and did not need the doctor.

November 11:
I went to the Arcadia Unit with an Australian pharmacist who was visiting with me. Mary was wandering the corridor as usual. Her mouth was again crusted so I asked for tooth paste and brush. With difficulty I got her teeth cleaned. Then I went looking for Jill Sobel and told her that I was worried that a man had attacked Mary on Friday evening. Jill said they would have to increase the man's medication. I escorted Mary to the dining room, and during dinner Mary became very aggressive putting her hands into a claw-like pose while snarling. Eventually I got her seated in the dining room and then joined my friend and we departed.

November 15:
I received a phone call from Manor Care about 11 a.m. to say that one of the men in the Arcadia Unit had pushed Mary and she had fallen backwards hitting her head on a door knob. It had caused a fairly large gash and she would have to go to the hospital emergency room for stitches. My Australian friends were still with me, so I was not able to take Mary to the hospital. Therefore I instructed them to send her in an ambulance and I phoned our daughter Elizabeth and asked her to join Mary in the hospital. After Elizabeth had returned her mother to Manor Care, she told me that her mother was "bright and seemed in good spirits". Elizabeth told me that she had read to Mary from a book she liked. Elizabeth went on to say that there were other people in both beds in Mary's room, also that the bathroom was quite dirty when she had returned with her mother. It is these frustrations that one has to contend with when a loved one is in a nursing

home. However, in general, the care was as good as could be expected and I do not believe that Mary was aware of these problems - she had even forgotten that the man had attacked her.

November 17:
On arriving at Manor Care I met with Tom Garvin, the Administrator, and pointed out to him that Mary needed to be better protected from the men who were attacking her. It then appeared that the man who had punched Mary in the nose on November 7th was not the same man who had pushed her down on the 15th. Tom said that they had the first man under control with drugs but the second man was quite aggressive and had attacked several other women. They were working with the psychiatrist and he was considering moving the man into a psychiatric hospital. Again this is an indication of the problems one faces, even in a relatively well-managed facility.

November 18:
In the mid-afternoon I received a call to say that Mary had fallen again. On further questioning, the attendant admitted that the same man had pushed her again. I then phoned Jill Sobel and she said that Mary had been screaming all the day and her behavior had upset the man and he attacked her, pushing her down. I said that I thought that Manor Care was going to place the man in a psychiatric hospital. Jill said that the psychiatrist had decided that he could be controlled with medication. I indicated that I was not pleased with the way they were handling the situation.

November 19:
There was another message that Mary had fallen again. I phoned Tom Garvin and he told me that the same man had pushed her, but Mary had not sustained further injuries. I also spoke with Jill and said that it is little wonder that Mary is agitated when men are attacking her and I asked that they do all they could to keep the men away from Mary. She said that the psychiatrist had placed the man on Haldol but that would take a few day to take effect. It had also been decided that if the man was not improved by Friday then he would be sent to a psychiatric hospital. She also said that it was not possible to keep Mary separated from the men.

November 24:

I received a call from Beth, one of the nurses at Manor Care, at 9:49 p.m. Mary had fallen again. I questioned Beth as to whether a man had pushed her. She assured me that she had not been pushed. In fact she said Mary just sank to the floor slowly.

December 2:

Call received about 10 a.m. to say that Mary had gone down in front of one of the attendants. She seemed to get twisted in her clothes and just went down gently. Again there was no injury. The caller asked me to pick up a prescription for her.

Approximately an hour later, Jill Sobel called to say that they thought Mary might have pneumonia and would I authorize them to have her x-rayed. I agreed. Then Jill said that if she had pneumonia she presumed I would not wish Mary to have antibiotics in accordance with my instructions. I said go ahead with the x-ray and I would then decide what to do. I thought I should discuss Mary's condition with her primary care physician, Dr. Perlstein, so I asked Jill to have him phone me after they had received the x-ray results.

I picked up the prescriptions and delivered them at about 5:35 p.m. Mary had finished dinner and while she felt hot as though she might have a fever she did not look too bad. I spoke with the nurse in charge and she confirmed that Mary had been x-rayed in the afternoon but they did not have the results. I asked her to let me know when they got the results. As I was walking out, I encountered Tom Garvin the Director. Again I mentioned that I would like to speak with Dr. Perlstein after they had the x-ray results. He said he would look into it in the morning.

At 7:41 p.m. Lavinia, the nurse on duty with whom I had spoken earlier, phoned to say they had the results but Mary had moved during the x-ray so they did not have a clear picture

December 3:

I spoke with Jill Sobel several times. First she said that there was evidence of fluid movement in the lungs. Later in the day she phoned to say that she had mis-read the x-ray report and what was said was that Mary had moved when they were taking the x-ray. She also said that Mary had a temperature of over 100 degrees. She was going to have Dr. Perlstein phone me. He did not phone me.

December 5:

I visited Mary at 12:10 p.m. One of the attendants was feeding her but I took over and gave her all her lunch. She did not appear to have a fever but she did have a hacking cough. I had intended to brush her teeth but decided that I did not want to get her cold so I left as soon as she finished her lunch.

Christmas Day:

I picked up Mary from the nursing home and with our younger daughter Marga-ret, who then lived in New York City, took her to the home of our elder daugh-ter, Elizabeth. The dinner went reasonably well although Mary did not seem to know what was going on and was quite restless.

December 29:

I received a phone call at 5:15 a.m. from Joan, the night nurse in the Arcadia unit, telling me that Mary had fallen out of bed. She had bruised her nose and had a gash in her forehead which was quite deep and bleeding a lot. Joan said she would call Dr. Perlstein since I had said that her doctor had to be notified before they sent her off to ER. About 15 minutes later Joan phoned back to say she spoke with the doctor on duty and he instructed them to send Mary to the Emergency room. At 7 a.m. Norristown Hospital phoned to seek my permission for them to treat Mary. I gave my O.K. and said I would be over in about an hour. At 7:30 Joan phoned to say they had put 9 stitches in Mary's forehead and that she was on her way back to Manor Care.

CHAPTER 20

MY NURSING HOME LOG – 1998

January 4:
I received a phone call about 3 p.m. to say Mary had fallen. I had previously been at Manor Care to feed Mary her lunch. She had been somewhat aggressive before lunch but had eaten well and let me clean her teeth. The attendant who called said she was lying on the floor and could not get up by herself but she did not seem to be injured.

January 12:
My secretary, Ruby, took a call from the nursing home to say that Mary had fallen out of bed onto the foam pad they now have beside her bed. She was not hurt but they planned to install a bed alarm which would go off when she fell out of bed.

January 14:
I received a call from Zara at about 9 p.m. to say Mary had fallen on her side while walking in the hall. Again she was not hurt. Zara was going to leave a message for the day shift to have the doctor reduce the tranquilizer from four tables per day to three.

January 26:
Jill Sobel, Director of the Arcadia Unit, phoned to ask permission for the "speech therapist" to review Mary's food intake. I asked why a speech therapist would be working on diet. Jill said that was the way they classified the work activities at Manor Care. I said "OK".

January 28:
When I arrived at the Arcadia Unit I found that Mary's food was chopped or pureed and her liquids were thickened to the level that I had to spoon them into her mouth.

February 2:
By this date, Mary was back to regular food and drink.

February 3:
The nurse on duty phoned to say that Mary had been terribly agitated all day. She would not allow anyone to touch her and she continued to walk and scream. I could hear Mary screaming over the phone. While I would have liked to go to see her it was just not possible that day.

February 4:
In light of yesterday's message that Mary was terribly agitated, I phoned Jill Sobel to discuss her condition. Jill said she was going to have the psychiatrist look at Mary.

February 5:
I phoned Jill in the morning to discuss the psychiatrist's findings. She said he had restored the Ativan back to four times per day. When I arrived at lunch time Mary was still very agitated. This was the first time that I was positively sure that she did not recognize me. She screamed continuously and was lashing out. Her behavior was upsetting the other patients.

February 6:
Elizabeth stopped by at lunch time and noted Mary's agitated state. This condition was persisting even though the nursing home was supposed to have returned Ativan doses to four times a day. I arrived at dinner time. She was still screaming and I stayed with her while the nurse on duty fed her in the hall way.

February 7:
In the morning I phoned Dr. Perlstein's office and discussed Mary's condition with the doctor's assistant. I suggested that she might be in pain but he said they

saw her almost every day and he did not think so. I then arrived at lunch time but she was too agitated to go into the dining room so I fed her off a mobile tray in the hall. Then I brushed her teeth. This time there was a major change in her. Up to this time she always would take the rinse water into her mouth and slush it round then spit it out. This time she just swallowed the water with the tooth paste. Since I had not cleaned her teeth for about a week her gums were bleeding more than usual.

February 16:
On this day, when I arrived at lunch time Mary was walking as usual. She brightened up and smiled when she saw me. We walked to the lunch room but after sitting for a while she became restless and started to bare her teeth and scream softly. I attempted to hold her still but she became more aggressive. Eventually the food arrived and I gave it to her, but her aggravation continued. Stephanie, the nurse on duty that day, seemed to become very protective of her.

February 18:
Again I called at lunch time. Mary was reasonable and ate everything on her tray. She also let me clean her teeth. About 9 p.m. Sarah phoned to say Mary had fallen again. She was trying to sit in a chair and missed it but she was O.K.

I went to Australia in March of 1998 and did not make another entry concerning incidents with Mary until July.

July 10:
Jennifer Poole, the new director of the Arcadia Unit, left a message on my voice mail that Mary had fallen and had a cut on her nose. It was not serious but Jennifer wanted to speak with me.

July 11:
The nurse on duty left a message on my voice mail this Saturday afternoon to say Mary had experienced a major fall and gashed her eye. The nurse had notified the doctor and had sent Mary to Norristown hospital by ambulance. But then the nurse called to tell me that Mary was back at the Arcadia Unit. It was not possible for me to go to the nursing home at that time and the nurse had indicated that Mary's condition was not serious.

July 12:

I went in for lunch on Sunday and found Elizabeth, and her husband Jim. Elizabeth was feeding Mary with both eyes black and four stitches on her right eyebrow. She was quiet but looked a mess. While there I was told that Jennifer Poole wanted me to phone her. She told me that there had been an outbreak of scabies and the other woman in Mary's room was infected, so Mary's clothes had been sent off to be laundered.

August 19:

I went to help with lunch but Mary was screaming so badly that there was little that I could do. I got her to lie on her bed but she continued to scream at the top of her lungs.

August 24:

When Elizabeth visited at supper time and fed Mary, Jennifer Poole told her that Mary had been screaming all afternoon. After she finished eating, Elizabeth took her mother to the room and found that she was wearing two right shoes so obviously her left foot was hurting. Moreover she found that Mary's right toe had lost most of the toe nail and was very red and swollen. By that time Jennifer had left so Elizabeth was not able to report the problems.

August 28:

I arrived at lunch time and found Mary on a bed in another room. I got her up and took her to the dining room. She ate everything without fuss. Then I got the nurse on duty to go to Mary's room with me and we took her shoes and stockings off. The nurse was surprised at how bad her toe was. She said she had no idea that Mary's foot was so bad. I asked how such a condition could go unnoticed. The nurse applied an antibiotic ointment and a band-aid. I asked that they have the podiatrist examine her.

October 22:

I received a voice message about noon to say that Mary had fallen. It was followed about 1:30 p.m. by a message from Tanya, a nurse who was particularly caring of Mary. Tanya's message was that Mary had a very bad cut in her forehead and they had sent her to the Emergency Room. As soon as I picked up these messages I went to Suburban General Hospital, where I arrived at about 4:30 p.m. I found Mary under sedation. The doctor in attendance told me that the gash on her forehead was so bad that they had to call for a plastic surgeon who was expected to arrive about 6 p.m. I sat with Mary who was connected to cardiac monitors.

She eventually started to come round from the sedation and commenced to scream uncontrollably. The cardiac monitor alarm went off a number of times as her pulse rate was varying from about 35 to over 100. Sometimes it stabilized at 63. She was receiving oxygen. One would have thought that the extreme screaming would have caused her heart to fail. As she continued to thrash about the wound started to bleed again. The nurse in attendance said she had lost pints of blood before I had arrived. The bandages which were removed while I was there were a sopping mess. At about 5 p.m. she was given more sedation as an intra-venous drip of Cephalin. The plastic surgeon arrived a little after 6 p.m. I was amazed to see that he had the stem of a candy sucker sticking out of his mouth. He did not look professional in any way.

For some reason they asked me to get them a copy of Mary's "Living Will", so I left for home to get a copy. When I returned, about 7:15 p.m., Mary had been admitted to the hospital on the 4th floor where I went to see her. At that stage she was again under sedation so I left. At about 10 a.m. on Friday I returned and found that she was again screaming but they had called for an ambulance to return her to the nursing home. I was able to calm her somewhat and she appeared to be sleeping when the ambulance arrived, so I followed the ambulance to Manor Care.

October 30:

The surgeon wanted to remove the stitches and insisted that we take Mary to his office in Suburban General Hospital. Tanya at Manor Care said they could remove the stitches. I decided that it was best for us to take Mary back to the surgeon so I phoned Elizabeth and asked if she could help me with Mary.

At the hospital a male volunteer got her into a wheel chair and we took her to the doctor's office with little trouble. While we were waiting Elizabeth arrived. Mary had been well sedated and there was little trouble in removing the stitches and returning her to the nursing home. The next day she was O.K. but on Sunday she was rather agitated.

November 2:

I was at a meeting in the morning when Tanya called and left a message that Mary had a "seizure". When I returned the call and spoke with Tanya she said Mary's eyes had gone very distant and she had been trembling. The doctor had been informed but she was resting quietly by the time I phoned.

November 3:

I went to see Mary in the evening. She was in a wheel chair and the nurse said she had not eaten at breakfast or lunch. However, I was able to get her to eat all the pizza provided for the evening meal. She drank juice and two little cartons of milk.

November 4:

This morning, I received a call from Tracy Acton who described herself as an "eating specialist." She said she had done an evaluation of Mary and found that she was having difficulty in chewing and swallowing. Consequently Tracy was ordering a puree diet and thickened beverages. She also wanted my permission to give Mary re-training to get her back on solid food. Tracy had contacted Aetna-U.S. Health Care for coverage for the cost of that procedure. I said I was not interested in trying to do that. If Mary could not eat that was that and I did not want to subject Mary to more problems. All we needed was for her to get liquid and be comfortable. She agreed. I pointed out that I had been able to get Mary to drink the previous evening and she had eaten all her pizza.

November 5:

Jennifer Poole, the director had phoned to say she wanted to see me. I arrived at lunch time and found Mary not only in a wheel chair but with a plastic covered foam cushion across the front of the chair to keep her in place.

The food service had sent up the normal meal with juice, milk, and hamburger. The helpers were concerned over this but I said I thought she could drink the juice. However, she could not. It ran out of her mouth. One of the attendants then put the thickening powder into the juice so it was the consistency of ice cream. She took both the juice and the milk as I fed them from a spoon. They also brought her a puree mixture. I was not able to identify what the food was but Mary ate it all.

That day I could not help thinking the end must be near. She had little color, a blank stare and had her mouth open most of the time. However, she did smile and laugh occasionally. Jennifer wanted me to sign an authorization for her to be restrained in the chair. She also said that Mary was no longer suitable for the Arcadia unit and if and when a bed became available in óne of the other units they wanted to move her. In fact it took almost two months for a bed to become available.

We visited Mary at Christmas but she was not in any condition to leave the nursing home..

CHAPTER 21

THE FINAL MONTHS 1999

February 4:

On this day Mary was transferred to the Valley Forge Unit of Manor Care. This is an intensive care facility which is not exclusively for Alzheimer's or dementia patients but includes others who were quite physically impaired. Here she was placed in a three person room but fortunately was in the bed closest to the window. When she needed to be moved she was placed in a large inclined chair.

On my arrival the nurse on duty, Fran, mentioned that the psychiatrist considered that Mary should be assigned to the Hospice program. For this to be granted, her primary care physician had to certify that she had less than 6 months to live.

I further investigated the hospice program and talked with Nancy Schertz the palliative care liaison person. She explained that Mary would remain a patient of Manor Care but that Caring Hospice Services would supplement her care with reimbursement through Medicare, Aetna-U.S Health Care

The supplementary services included a weekly visit by their doctor, three visits per week by an RN and daily visits by a **social worker.**

February 15:

I arrived shortly after lunch and was told that there had been a problem with Mary almost choking on the thickened liquid they were feeding her. When I arrived she was lying in bed on her side and a fluid was slowly coming out of her open mouth. She did not open her eyes and seemed quite out of it. By this stage her mouth was almost always open and she was breathing in gasps.

February 22:

Both Elizabeth and I arrived in the early afternoon and Mary was in the big reclining chair. They said she had eaten well. Elizabeth and I then took her for a walk round the corridors. She seemed reasonable and laughed at something we said.

The next four months were somewhat uneventful. Either Elizabeth or I tried to visit the nursing home nearly every day and help with a meal. On nice days we wheeled Mary out into the sun on the patio.

June 6:

I was not informed that Mary had had two Grand Mal seizures. I only learned about them when I phoned Dr. Pearlstein on Monday to ask about a lumbar tap which I wanted for Dr. Balin. He would use the spinal fluid to determine if Mary was infected with *Chlamydia pneumoniae*. Dr. Pearlstein told me that, since Mary had experienced the seizures, she would be eligible to have the tap taken at the hospital and insurance would pay.

June 8:

I arrived at Suburban General Hospital at 9:30 a. m. and completed registration for Mary. Elizabeth had gone to Manor Care and was to follow the ambulance. Dr. Pearlstein came up for the procedure. Mary did not seem too traumatized by the procedure. Elizabeth had bought a cheese burger but it was soon apparent that Mary had no chance of eating it. She did have some food and thick drink. One of the nurses in the Valley Forge Unit, Charlene Calhoun, took great care of Mary. One day she said to me, "Mary must have been a special woman. I am very impressed by how her daughter comes to take care of her. Very few of the other patients have family members who take such interest and care of them.

July 6:

Charlene Calhoun phoned to say that Mary had not eaten for the past two days and was very agitated. When I arrived about lunch time Mary was screaming and thrashing about. Charlene phoned Dr. Perlstein and he prescribed Morphine 2 ml to be given under the tongue every 15 to 20 minutes. Charlene gave her one dose but that was the only dose available in the Valley Forge Unit. Charlene then tried to borrow another dose of morphine from one of the other units but as Mary had calmed down following that first dose, the senior nurse in the Valley Forge unit would not approve it.

July 7:

In the morning I contacted Charlene at the Valley Forge unit and found that Mary was again very agitated. I then conferred with both our daughters. Elizabeth said she was leaving for the nursing home and Margaret said she would take a train from New York immediately. We also decided to contact St. David's Church. The Associate priest, Rev. Rudy Moore, who had known Mary for years, said he would go to the nursing home and give Mary "Last Rites".

I drove to Manor Care and met Elizabeth who was already there. Mary was restless and screaming intermittently. I then phoned Dr. Pearlstein. He was annoyed that his order of the day before had not been carried out and Mary should not have been in such obvious pain. He then spoke with Charlene and repeated his orders for Mary to be given 2ml. morphine sub-lingual every 15 to 20 minutes.

We decided to withhold treatment until after Rev. Moore arrived at about 11:30 a.m. He then proceeded to give Last Rites as prescribed in the Episcopal Book of Common Prayer. Elizabeth and I were present but Margaret had not yet arrived from New York.

After Rev. Moore left, Charlene started doses of morphine. Mary continued to scream for some time. Margaret arrived about 1:30 p.m. It was obvious that Mary was unable to swallow and was in considerable pain. Approximately 10 doses of morphine were administered and Mary was continuing to scream. Margaret and I went for some supper about 6 p.m. and when we returned Mary was sleeping quietly.

At approximately 7:30 p.m. Mary stopped breathing and the nurse checked that her heart had stopped.

One of the attendants thought so much of Mary that she had volunteered to stay for a second shift instead of going off at 3 pm, so that she could be with Mary when she died. That woman then attended to Mary and had her dressed and her hair done.

That was the last time we saw Mary. I phoned the University of Pennsylvania so her body could be taken there for the autopsy.

My life with Mary was over.

LIFE WITHOUT MARY

CHAPTER 22

IN MEMORIAM

Arrangements for Mary's funeral had been put in place in March of 1987, so now it was largely a matter of up-dating some of the details. We had a burial plot in the grave yard surrounding St. David's Church.

The church was built by Welsh settlers in 1715 and our grave site was some 50 yards from the original building among a stand of old trees. Some of the surrounding graves were of soldiers who died during the Revolutionary war. It is certainly a beautiful and peaceful place as described in a Longfellow poem, ***Old St. David's at Radnor,*** written when he visited in March of 1880:

> *"What an image of peace and rest*
> *Is this little church among its graves!*
> *All is so quiet; the troubled breast,*
> *The wounded spirit, the heart oppressed,*
> *Here may find the repose it craves."*

Mary died on Wednesday July 7, 1999. In order for some people to reach Philadelphia it was decided to hold the burial service on Monday July 11. The Reverend Frank Allen, the Rector of St. David's Church led the service and Rev. Rudolph Moore gave the Eulogy. We had decided on the full Episcopal service with the Eucharist, and the closed casket was in the church for the service and covered with a plain shroud. We had requested that instead of flowers, mourners should make donations to the Alzheimer's Association in Mary's name.

During the Eulogy, the Rev. Moore recited the following:

Poem at Point of Death

I thought I heard her say,
"I'll be leaving you today
When the priest brought last rites
I knew I'd see the lights
And the splendid sights of my Father's house
I stand at God's door and wave goodbye
But I really don't want to hear you cry
For what's past.
It's past and the present is prologue

Don't weep for the past
Or what didn't last
But weep for the love
I couldn't help shrug,
And the lack of choice,
And the loss of voice
There was so much I still had to say.
I don't want to hear you cry
For days gone by
The past is past and the present is prologue.
I'll be leaving you today. That's what I heard her say

EPILOGUE...

Is Heritage a Factor?

Eventually I heard from Dr. Christopher Clark the director of the Memory Disorders Clinic at the University of Pennsylvania where Mary's brain had been lodged. Dr. Clark said that her brain was one of the more interesting ones they had looked at and he expected that they might have up to three years of work on it. He asked again if Mary was descended from the "Volga River Germans". In view of that question we initiated further investigation of Mary's ancestry.

Mary's grandmother and grandfather on her mother's side had emigrated from England and her mother was the first in her family to be born in the United States. We knew that her father was born in Wisconsin and it was always assumed that his family had come from Berlin. However, on closer investigation it was found that his mother had been adopted and since adoption records in those years were closed it is impossible to say where she had come from but it must be assumed that she was German. Mary's German Grandfather and Grandmother had been married in Wisconsin in the later 1880s.

Because of Dr. Clark's question about the Volga River Germans I undertook further investigation. From a historical point of view, Catherine the Great who became Czarina of Russia on the death of her husband was originally a German Princess. In the 1760s two events occurred that resulted in a number of German settlers moving to villages on the Volga River in Russia. First there had been a recession in Germany and many farmers had fallen on bad times. Also, the area along the Volga River was very sparsely settled and the Tartars had been marauding in the region. Therefore Catherine contacted some of her friends in Germany and asked that German farmers be settled in the area. In return for migrating Catherine made several commitments to them: They were exempted from serving in the Russian Army and they did not have to pay Russian taxes.

Sometime after arrival in Russia one German experienced a mutation on the first chromosome. This mutation was such that it causes those who inherited it to develop Alzheimer's disease, usually at an early age. Naturally this gene mutation was passed on to the descendents of the person in whom the mutation had first occurred. In a relatively brief period quite a number of individuals in several villages were carrying the gene.

About 100 years after the first Germans went to Russia, Catherine's promises were rescinded, taxes were levied and the Germans were drafted into the Russian Army. As a result many of these people decided to migrate again - this time to the United States - some ending up in Kansas and Eastern Washington State. Several researchers at the University of Washington in Seattle noted that many of the descendents of these people were developing Alzheimer's disease at a relatively early age. As a consequence, several papers were written by Schellenburger and Bird which reported this unusual incidence of the disease.

Now it happens that while Mary's great grandmother had gone to Wisconsin from Berlin, it was known that she had been an orphan. As there was a possibility that the great grandmother may have been descended from the Volga River Germans I discussed the situation with some at the Penn Memory Center and they sent a sample of her DNA to the University of Washington. They determined that she was not one of those who had inherited the faulty gene.

A Promising Theory

One of the first "Caregiver" meetings I attended was at a major Philadelphia suburban hospital. The doctor making the presentation stressed that Alzheimer's disease is a **neurological disease** and not a **psychological disease.** I believe that this is an important distinction.

There are many processes which cause degeneration in mental health. One is physical injury; another is a chemical imbalance which leads to conditions such as schizophrenia and many other physiological conditions. Such conditions include a deterioration of the blood circulation in the brain - stroke being the most common, genetic diseases such as Down syndrome and Huntington's disease, and diseases which lead to degeneration of nerve cells. Alzheimer's disease is characterized by the deposition of a protein substance known as *amyloid protein* throughout the cerebral cortex. The deposition of amyloid protein is somewhat analogous to the deposition of cholesterol in blood vessels. The deposits of amyloid protein interrupt the flow of nerve impulses between different parts of the brain and eventually lead to destruction of cells. A very closely related disease is Pick's disease in which cell atrophy is confined to the frontal and temporal lobes of the brain.

While psychiatrists are sometimes called on to treat the clinical symptoms of Alzheimer's disease, it appears that most current research on the disease is being performed by neurologists working in a number of leading universities and hospitals throughout the world. A listing of these research centers can be found on the Alzheimer's Web Page http://www.alzweb.org

Much of the current research is involved in examining factors which might lead to the development of Alzheimer's disease. There is some evidence that hereditary factors may have a role in the susceptibility to the disease. Three gene alterations are more common in persons who develop Alzheimer's disease. The ApoE4 gene on chromosome 19 seems to be linked to the most common form of Alzheimer's disease, that known as *Late Onset*. There are changes in genes on chromosomes 14 and 21 which appear to be more common in persons who develop Alzheimer's disease in early or middle age, a condition termed *Early Onset*. At present it does not appear that Alzheimer's disease is specifically inherited.

Other research is looking at the role of Tau Protein. Tau is a protein found in the walls of cells. When the cell dies and breaks down then this protein is included in the tangles which are typically found in the brains of persons who have died with Alzheimer's disease.

The clinical symptoms of Alzheimer's disease have been extensively described (they certainly vary from individual to individual) and the pathological conditions of the brains of persons who have died from Alzheimer's disease are well documented. As good as this research is there are still very significant gaps in our knowledge of the cause of Alzheimer's disease. What specific mechanism causes the amyloid protein plaques and tangles to develop? Does the amyloid protein cause the degeneration of the nerve cells? Or do the accumulations result from some other mechanism?

One of my professional colleagues was Dr. James Prior, a microbiologist who served as an adjunct professor at the Philadelphia College of Osteopathic Medicine. Dr Prior, knowing of my wife's condition put me in touch with Dr. Brian Balin a member of the faculty at the Philadelphia College of Osteopathic Medicine. Dr. Balin was previously working at Allegheny University of the Health Sciences formerly known as the Medical College of Pennsylvania and Hahnemann University. When Allegheny University suffered financial difficulties and declared bankruptcy, Dr. Balin moved to the Philadelphia College of Osteopathic Medicine. Dr. Balin is an experimental neuropathologist with a background in microbiology who, at one time, had a connection with the Memory Disorders Clinic at the University of Pennsylvania. In a limited study, Dr. Balin observed that an autopsy of brains of some patients who died from Alzheimer's disease revealed an infection with the bacteria *Chlamydia pneumoniae*.

The results of Dr. Balin's research are published in Medical Microbiology and Immunology (1998) Vol: 187, pages 23-42. This study looked at the presence of the bacteria in post-mortem brain samples from patients with and without late-onset Alzheimer's disease. The presence of bacteria was determined by a very sensitive test known as the polymerase chain reaction (PCR) assay for DNA sequences from the bacterium. Using this test, Dr. Balin and his associates were able to show that brain areas with typical Alzheimer's disease related neuropathology were infected with *Chlamydia pneumoniae* in 17 out of 19 patients.

Similar analysis of identical brain areas of 18 out of another 19 who were presumed not to have suffered from Alzheimer's disease, were PCR negative, that is, no bacteria were present. As a further check, electron-microscopic studies (that allow one to view inside of cells) of tissues from brains of persons affected by Alzheimer's disease also revealed the presence of the bacteria. In contrast to this, the electron-microscopic studies of brains from persons who had not died from Alzheimer's disease failed to identify any bacteria.

It is unfortunate that this initial research was limited to a total of only 38 persons, although subsequent studies by Dr. Balin and others have continued to find evidence for this infection in Alzheimer's disease. Dr. Balin's research has received NIH and Alzheimer's Foundation funding in the past, but currently his studies are not funded through these organizations. Dr. Balin's work is controversial in the field of Alzheimer's disease and has been criticized by others, especially neurologists, working on the study of this disease. This criticism by persons working in one field of medicine of persons working on novel concepts and in interdisciplinary fields is not uncommon and it may even occur between researchers in the same field. In 1983 Barry Marshall, an Australian doctor, discovered that the bacterium *Helicobacter pylori* is the cause of most stomach ulcers. Not only did the medical profession in Australia totally discount Dr. Marshall's work but when he came to the United States the medical profession in general laughed off his theory and the American Society of Gastroenterologists declared that it was just not possible for bacteria to cause ulcers. It is amazing that it took almost 12 years for the medical profession to accept the truth of Dr. Marshall's work and treat ulcer patients for the bacteria.

An article by Philip Ross in the November, 1999 issue of Forbes Magazine reviews the research which has indicated that a number of diseases which were thought to have various causes may actually be the result of bacterial infection. Ross states that bacteria and other organisms such as viruses have been proven to be the root cause of ulcers, stomach cancer, liver cancer, Burkett's Lymphoma, cervical cancer, and oral cancer. In addition he indicated that living organisms (bacteria and/or viruses) are suspected to be contributing agents in atherosclerosis, Alzheimer's disease, multiple sclerosis, juvenile diabetes, asthma, non-melanoma skin cancer, and colon cancer.

Why do the neurologists fail to recognize the possibility that bacteria may in fact be at least a contributing factor in the development of Alzheimer's disease? One of the reasons is that most neurologists are not necessarily well trained in microbiology and other disciplines. On one occasion when I mentioned to Dr. Parr that *Chlamydia pneumoniae* may be a contributing factor in the occurrence of Alzheimer's disease he responded that such a concept was nonsense. You will recall that Justin Parr was the doctor who first recognized that Mary may have Alzheimer's disease and he is well versed in geriatric and degenerative diseases. He went on to say that the brains of persons who died with Alzheimer's disease have been studied for a long time and that if bacteria were present they would have been seen years ago. On referring that statement to Dr. Balin he indicated that one of the problems that others in the medical profession have in recognizing *Chlamydia pneumoniae* is that the organism is intracellular and so small. *Chlamydia pneumoniae* is exceedingly small (0.2-0.4 µm) that is approximately in the same size range as some viruses. Thus these bacteria can only be seen under an electron microscope or with specific antibodies that label the organism within cells. The way in which a positive identification is obtained is by the PCR test as used by Dr. Balin in the study reported above.

As the NIH funds for Dr. Balin's work were discontinued a group of people have formed a non-profit foundation to help the work to continue. This is the *Foundation for Research into Diseases of Aging* (FRIDA). The purpose of this tax exempt foundation is to receive donations from wealthy individuals or corporations and distribute it to the laboratory headed by Dr. Balin so that he may continue his novel studies.

Following newspaper articles and radio interviews, Dr. Balin received calls from spouses of several persons suffering from Alzheimer's disease. In some of these cases, Dr. Balin worked with the patient's primary care physician and was able to show that the Alzheimer's sufferer was carrying *C. pneumoniae* in their spinal fluid. It was then recommended that the patient be given azithromycin (brand name Zithromax). In several of these cases the patients showed improvement of their dementia.

One particular case with which I had personal knowledge was the wife of one of the men in the group which met together in Philadelphia for monthly luncheons and to share experience related to caring for our spouses. When this man heard of Dr. Balin's research he arranged for his wife to give a specimen of spinal fluid. On examination of this specimen by Dr. Balin's laboratory it was determined that the woman was infected with *C. pneumonia*. Her primary care physician then prescribed Zithromax.

After his wife had been on the drug for several months he was ecstatic. Apparently his wife had been virtually unable to speak for a year or more but since taking the Zithromax she was speaking quite clearly. Also she was discussing what she would like for her birthday. For several years she had been quite unaware of her birthday.

In a discussion with Dr. Balin in late 1999 he told me that his laboratory had been able to show that when a culture of *C. pneumonia* was added to growing brain cells, the cells were killed and amyloid protein was released.

In spite of the criticism from neurologists, Dr. Balin has continued his study of bacteria in the brains of persons suffering with Alzheimer's disease. In August of 2013 he sent me copies of six research studies which have been published in various scientific journals. Some twenty two scientists had co-authored these papers.

Not only has this work been published in American scientific journals but one was published in the journal of the Federation of European Microbiological Scientists. All of these research papers describe how *Chlamydia pneumoniae* has been detected in the brains, or spinal fluid, of persons who have been confirmed to have had Alzheimer's disease. Bacteria have not been detected in control groups who do not have Alzheimer's disease.

Over 200 pharmaceutical products have been developed and tested in phase three clinical trials but so far only 5 have received approval from the FDA. All of these products are designed to chemically improve the communication between brain cells - that is they work at the synapses. The jury is still out on this theory but the research continues.

For more detail on the research by Dr. Brian Balin and others, log on to pubmed.com, enter *Balin BJ* in the search window to gain access to recent studies such as the six listed here:

Immunohistological detection of Chlamydia pneumoniae in the **Alzheimer's disease** brain.

Hammond CJ, Hallock LR, Howanski RJ, Appelt DM, Little CS, Balin BJ.
BMC Neurosci. 2010 Sep 23;11:121. doi: 10.1186/1471-2202-11-121.
Toward a unifying hypothesis in the development of Alzheimer's disease.
Balin B, Abrams JT, Schrogie J.
CNS Neurosci Ther. 2011 Dec;17(6):587-9. doi: 10.1111/j.1755-5949.2011.00269

Chlamydophila pneumoniae and the etiology of late-onset Alzheimer's disease.

Balin BJ, Little CS, Hammond CJ, Appelt DM, Whittum-Hudson JA, Gérard HC, Hudson AP.

J Alzheimers Dis. 2008 May;13(4):371-80.

Chlamydophila (Chlamydia) pneumoniae in the Alzheimer's brain.

Gérard HC, Dreses-Werringloer U, Wildt KS, Deka S, Oszust C, Balin BJ, Frey WH 2nd, Bordayo EZ, Whittum-Hudson JA, Hudson AP.

FEMS Immunol Med Microbiol. 2006 Dec;48(3):355-66. Epub 2006 Oct 18.

Chlamydia pneumoniae induces Alzheimer-like amyloid plaques in brains of BALB/c mice.

Little CS, Hammond CJ, MacIntyre A, Balin BJ, Appelt DM.

Neurobiol Aging. 2004 Apr;25 (4):419-29.

Evaluation of CSF-Chlamydia pneumoniae, CSF-tau, and CSF-Abeta42 in Alzheimer's disease and vascular dementia.

Paradowski B, Jaremko M, Dobosz T, Leszek J, Noga L.

J Neurol. **2007** Feb; 25 4(2):154-9. Epub **2007** Feb 21.

Acknowledgments

I am grateful to the following contributors for their help in bringing our family's experience with Alzheimer's Disease to fruition:

Jim Cassidy for his suggestions regarding the structure and continuity of the story;

Jeanne Scarpato Kysela, for her concept and creation of the front cover: I immediately liked the mirror image of the title because this disease turns life upside down for the patient and has tremendous impact on the caregivers;

Francis X. Feeney for his time and expertise in enhancing all our photographs; Frank took 40 and 50 year old images and made them look like new; in addition, Frank enhanced and fine-tuned front and back covers;

Dr. Brian Balin for his tireless research into the possible connection between the bacteria *Chlamydia pneumonia* and Alzheimer's Disease;

My thanks to all,

Philip C. Minter, AM

www.ingramcontent.com/pod-product-compliance
Lightning Source LLC
Chambersburg PA
CBHW040807200526
45159CB00022B/37